PREGNANT AND ALONE
How You Can Help an Unwed Friend

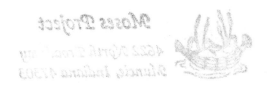

Other books in the *Heart and Hand* Series:

CAREGIVING: When Someone You Love Grows Old
John Gillies

FRIENDSHIP UNLIMITED: How You Can Help a Disabled Friend
Joni Eareckson Tada with Bev Singleton

SPLITTING UP: When Your Friend Gets a Divorce
Dandi Daley Knorr

WHEN YOUR FRIEND GETS CANCER: How You Can Help
Amy Harwell with Kristine Tomasik

PREGNANT & ALONE

How you can help
an unwed friend

Henrietta VanDerMolen

Harold Shaw Publishers
Wheaton, Illinois

The *Heart and Hand* Series

Cover photo © 1989 by Jim Whitmer

ISBN 0-87788-707-1

Library of Congress Cataloging-in-Publication Data
VanDerMolen, Henrietta.
    Pregnant and alone : how you can help an unwed friend / Henrietta VanDerMolen.
        p. cm. — (Heart and hand series)
        Bibliography: p.
        ISBN 0-87788-707-1 :
        1. Unmarried mothers—Care—United States. 2. Teenage mothers—Care—United States. I. Title. II. Series.
HV700.5.V36   1989
362.8'392—dc19   89-5955
                                                                    CIP

98 97 96 95 94 93 92 91 90 89

10 9 8 7 6 5 4 3 2 1

Be not forgetful to entertain strangers:
for thereby some have entertained angels unawares.
Hebrews 13:2, KJV

This book is gratefully dedicated
to "Sandy,"
the first pregnant girl who lived with me,
who was indeed my "unaware angel,"
to Dr. Jim and Virginia,
who helped set my feet in this pathway of service,
and to Jeff,
whose role of sensitive and concerned "brother"
was so important to the girls who lived with us.

A few years ago I found myself pregnant, scared, and virtually alone. I couldn't keep my child, and my parents didn't want me to.

Shortly after, I went to stay with Henrietta, a wonderful Christian lady. It amazed me that a woman would accept me, *single*, pregnant, and alone, into her home—then I found out she'd been doing that for many girls just like me!

I won't say I could never have made it without Henrietta, but I will say she's the best friend I had at the time. She prayed for me, and she was beside me when I needed a friend. It took a lot of pain, suffering, and sleepless nights to decide to give my baby up for adoption. It still hurts, but throughout my time with Henrietta, she helped me see that I was doing a beautiful thing by giving life—a child—to someone who needed and wanted a baby, a family aching for a child. I feel good about the choice I made. Henrietta made me feel special when I thought I was a nobody.

I hope another girl in trouble will be touched by her warm heart and strong faith in God.

A birth mother

Contents

Foreword

I wish a book like this were not needed. But the fact remains that pregnancies of unmarried women are epidemic in the United States with no sign of abating. A large number of cases I see in my courtroom on a daily basis include women—mostly teens—who are pregnant and unmarried.

Resisting the temptation to preach moralistically at women who become pregnant outside of wedlock, Henrietta VanDerMolen has rolled up her sleeves and really *done something* to show God's love to these women. I'm reminded of our Lord's gracious response both to the woman at the well with her succession of husbands and boyfriends and to the other woman caught in adultery. Without compromising the truth, Jesus lovingly met all people—whether notorious sinners or not—at the point of their unique need.

This certainly is what Henrietta VanDerMolen has done with her life. I've had the privilege of knowing Henrietta personally for many years. Even while her husband was alive and she was very busy raising her six children, Henrietta was a dynamo of love and concern for others. But you would think that with the passing of her beloved husband and the exodus of her children to homes of their own, Henrietta would join the legion of "Condo Commandos" and begin a life of ease in some sunny clime. Not so. When confronted with the pressing needs of her "first" unwed mother, Henrietta, prompted by the Spirit of God, literally jumped at the opportunity to help.

Since that first opportunity, Henrietta has opened her heart and home to more than thirty young women in need who have been able to share the burden of their challenging pregnancies with her. Invigorated by the joy of serving and educated well by the experience, Henrietta now writes this book to help us learn to follow her example in our own way when we are confronted, as we all sooner or later will be, with a friend or relative who finds herself pregnant out of wedlock. Ignoring the problem or turning our backs on these women ("They got into this mess; let them get out of it by themselves!") is not a godly response. In hating the sin for the evil it brings on the sinner and others, we can and should learn to love the woman, helping her (and the father of the child, to the extent possible) to experience the healing that God alone can bring, often through people like you and me.

Sex is a wonderful, marvelous creation of an all-wise God. While man's sinfulness has corrupted this creation in many ways, God still uses sexuality to create unique children to continue the human race and to accomplish his ultimate purposes in this world. With God, there are no accidents. He is involved in the conception of *every* child, whether conceived by wedded parents or not. Life is not primarily biological; it exists under the infinite sovereignty of God, who alone creates people in the womb. When a young woman becomes pregnant through a rape, we instinctively recoil in disgust and tend to gravitate toward abortion, as if killing the unborn child somehow expiates the crime of the rapist. But as Henrietta reminds us, the precious child thus created still bears the image of his or her Creator. Abortion, therefore, is not the truly just response to a rape-induced pregnancy. While relatively few crisis pregnancies occur as a result of rape (approximately 1 percent), they still do happen, and we need to be prepared to offer our help.

For the vast majority of cases, however, the woman voluntarily has engaged in immorality and becomes pregnant. While these situations engender far less natural sympathy in us, we are still in the right to follow Henrietta's lead by offering our assistance and direction to help lead these women back on the track—for their sakes and the sake of their children.

Sin always produces deadly consequences. Prevention is far better than trying to perform damage control. Clearly we must exert much more effort at pointing more forcefully with our lives at the need for individual, familial, and societal morality. But until our sex-crazed culture moves closer to the standards of biblical morality, we will need to listen ever more intently to the counsel of Henrietta VanDerMolen, learning from her words and life how better to reach out in love to those suffering from the ravages of their own conduct and helping them to steer their lives back to safety and wholeness. As believers, we can do no less.

Hon. Randall J. Hekman
Grand Rapids, Michigan

Special thanks

to my editor Annette, who put the polish and pizzazz on
   everything;
to the editorial director at Shaw, Ramona, whose editing,
   encouragement, and writing tips were invaluable;
to my friends at Evangelical Child & Family Agency,
   who gave such good advice: Doris, Donna, Eleanor,
   and Cindy;
and to my granddaughter Alyssa, who deciphered my
   scribbles and put them on computer.

Introduction

One lovely day in the spring of 1981, Dr. Jim, a local obstetrician, called my daughter Virginia to ask if she could house and counsel a pregnant girl. Sandy* was coming from out of state to be under Dr. Jim's care. Since Virginia was a pyschologist and was busy with a six-month-old baby, Dr. Jim thought the arrangement might be mutual—help with the kids in exchange for a loving home and some counseling. But Virginia had her hands full with her two older children, and their house had no guest room.

"Let me ask my mom," she suggested to Dr. Jim. "She lives next door and has room. If she agrees, I could counsel the girl."

I had never considered having pregnant girls living with me, and it certainly didn't seem appropriate at that point. At the time, my youngest son—the only one left at home of my six children—had just turned seventeen and was a junior in high school. How would Jeff react? Would he be embarrassed? Friendly? How would he be influenced by this "naughty" girl? My protective mother's heart was concerned about his last few years at home. Jeff's dad died when he was thirteen, and these last few years had been hard for Jeff and me as we went through that separation together. We were close friends. I certainly didn't want to jeopard-

*names have been changed to protect privacy

ize that relationship, and I didn't want him to be uncomfortable in his own home.

I pondered and prayed over the decision, and finally decided it would be best to go straight to him for his reaction.

"Jeff," I began, "we have a door of opportunity and service before us, but I don't know if we should open it. I can't decide whether to walk through it or reconsider it a few years from now. We've been asked to make a home for a pregnant girl for the next four or five months. I'm interested, but I'm concerned about you. I don't want you to feel uncomfortable here, and I don't want your friends to feel embarrassed to come over. Do you want to think it over?"

"Go for it, Mom," Jeff said, without missing a beat. His response was firm and enthusiastic. "We'll all handle it okay."

"Great! Since we're both against abortion, this seems like a practical way to put some wheels under our convictions." I smiled. I should have known.

Making Room for Sandy

Before Sandy arrived, I learned that she was twenty-one and had finished two years of college. To my relief, I didn't think she would be interested in a seventeen-year-old high schooler—he would be "safe" no matter what her influence. (My mother's instincts were working overtime again. Oh, Sandy, I apologize! I had never met you then!)

But Sandy was a darling! Everyone loved her, and she spent many hours next door receiving counseling from Virginia and helping with my grandchildren. She moved into the efficiency apartment attached to my home and chose to stay there and do her own cooking. She brought in her own sewing machine and sewed for herself and for others. Since she was planning to release her baby for adoption, she made a beautiful quilt to send with her baby, which she designed and embroidered herself. Her mother, sister, and father all came from out of state to visit her at different times during those months.

Sandy had been through a terrible time with Ron, her fiancé. The wedding date was set, the dress purchased, the preparations made, and the invitations stamped and addressed, when Ron's father had a talk with his son. According to certain common property laws in the state they lived in, half of everything Ron owned would become Sandy's when they married. Ron couldn't accept such a "loss," and he broke their engagement. Sandy was devastated, and her family was hurt and surprised as well. Why did that wealthy father wait so long to discuss these financial matters with Ron? And was Ron too shallow and money-hungry to share? Did he really love her?

Although their engagement was broken, Sandy continued to see her boyfriend. Ron began to pressure her to have sexual relations with him, although they never had before. Sandy yearned to win him back to his previous commitment and wanted to show how much she loved him, so she gave in *one time*. That was all it took; Sandy became pregnant.

Sandy and Ron were both college students but on different campuses. They began suspecting that Sandy was pregnant, and once the pregnancy was confirmed, Sandy never heard from him again, although Ron did have contact with an attorney. When the spring quarter ended, she came to live with Jeff and me. In the months that followed, Ron never called her parents to ask how or where Sandy was. When the attorney handling the case called him to inform him of the baby's birth, Ron's first question was, "Boy or girl?"

"It isn't important for you to know," the attorney answered him.

"Well, who does it look like?" was his second question.

The attorney replied, "Since I've never seen you or the baby, I really cannot answer your question."

Ron never asked about Sandy. The attorney requested that Ron sign one of the two documents he had been sent—one accepted his paternity but released the child for adoption; the other denied paternity.

"I plan to pursue a political career, and I can't have this on my record. I'm denying paternity."

His answer was the last in a long line of rejections—a broken engagement promise, abandonment during pregnancy, disinterestedness in Sandy's physical or emotional health after the birth, and denial of paternity.

Sandy's mom, a lovely lady, came to share with and support Sandy during the baby's birth. She was the first—but certainly not the last!—grandmother who cried on my shoulder as she watched her first grandchild going out of her life.

Sandy named her baby "David," after the king whose sexual sin was forgiven by God. She hoped her child would also someday be "a man after God's own heart."

What Next?

My experience with Sandy was wonderful! I knew I had to go on being involved with single pregnant young women, but I also realized that if I waited for another referral from a local doctor, it would be a long wait. So I contacted Evangelical Child and Family Agency, a local agency, to make my home available. The agency took me through their state licensing procedure, the police check, the finger printing, reference checks, conferences, and inspection of my home. The process was very thorough, taking several months. Since then, my license has been renewed every two years.

Why? My main concern and growing love has been for the girls! I want to provide a loving and non-judgmental environment in which a girl can await the birth of her baby, knowing she will be well nourished for her own health's sake and for the health of the baby and that she will receive good counseling to help her with the decisions she is facing. I also hope to challenge a young woman to seek a better direction for her future.

Perhaps sheltering two or three girls a year doesn't seem to make a dent in the vast problem of teenage pregnancy. My agency alone worked with 180 girls from two states last year. There is quite a number of foster homes, but there is almost always a need for more. Your open home may not seem to you to make a significant difference to such an overwhelming national crisis, but it does. And it makes a world of difference to those young women!

How glad I am that I climbed out of my comfortable, complacent rut to meet girls where and when they are hurting and facing a very tough situation. Their lives and experiences have taught me so much; I am a more compassionate woman for having known them.

Now It's Happening to You

A friend of yours (or maybe your daughter, granddaughter, sister, or niece) just came to you in tears and told you, "I think I'm pregnant!"—and she is not married. Her news stopped you cold.

"I never would have guessed . . ."

"I'm so disappointed in her . . ."

"I feel sick . . ."

Maybe your first thought was one of these. Maybe the emotions came so thick and fast that you couldn't seem to sort them out.

Whether you respond with shock, with anger, with tears, or with gentleness, sooner or later the questions come down to: "What do I do now? What am *I* supposed to do with this information? How can I help?"

Help!

When your friend shared her painful secret with you, she made a direct claim on your friendship. The kind of friendship she's hoping to receive from you is more than just a let's-go-shopping-together-on-the-weekends or a come-on-over-for-a-cup-of-tea friendship. Your friend is saying, "Be there for me. Bear this burden with me!"

Maybe—probably—you feel unequal to meet such a need, to weather such a crisis with your friend. Don't give up before you ever begin! There are many ways you can help—by listening, praying, learning about your friend's options, and even by providing some counsel.

What It's All About

Right now you are facing a ministry challenge: the challenge of being a true friend to a young woman in crisis. That's what this book is all about. The coming chapters will encourage you in the difficult role of listener/supporter/counselor, offer guidelines and necessary information, and steer you clear of some of the pitfalls.

Your heart may feel heavy with concern for your unmarried, pregnant friend right now. The information in this book may help both of you sort through the deluge of choices your friend is facing. Ask God now to help you be the best loving and supportive friend you can be!

Henrietta VanDerMolen

1

Getting Started

Consider this scenario: Your best friend has just told you that she thinks she is pregnant. She has missed her period, and she feels different—very sleepy and a little nauseous. She's panicking. So far only you and she know her fears.

Don't panic! Encourage your friend to purchase an at-home pregnancy testing kit from the drugstore. Although they are not 100 percent accurate, they are fairly reliable and easy to use. If your friend feels comfortable with going to a local Crisis Pregnancy Center, she can have an accurate test there. She may want you to go with her.

If the test indicates that your friend is pregnant, as she suspected, you can help her make a plan for telling her folks, absorbing all the information about her various options, and for doing what's best for that unborn child.

First Things First

The best place to begin is with prayer. Pray for your friend, and pray for yourself! God's Word advises, "If any of you lacks wisdom, he should ask God, who gives generously to all without finding fault, and it will be given to him" (James 1:5).

Start with prayer, and don't stop praying!

Your Friend's Heartache

When you discover that your friend is pregnant, try to put aside your own shock and disappointment and concentrate on your friend's needs. At this point, probably one of the last things your friend needs is to be reminded that sex outside of marriage is wrong and foolish and dishonoring to God. Often she is already well aware of those facts! You can communicate your loving help and support without communicating approval of her poor choices.

Your friend is facing one dilemma—the dilemma of her pregnancy—but many, many choices. She has so many elements bombarding her—herself, her family, her boyfriend, you, her future, the child's future, etc.—that she probably will have a hard time thinking about one thing at a time or keeping one emotion separate from another. Be prepared to help her think and to help her *feel*. Be prepared to share her emotions. Be prepared to be patient with her distress.

When a girl's pregnancy has been confirmed by a doctor's visit, she usually enters a period of emotional turmoil, a period of denial, anger, fear, and panic. These statements reflect the various stages of this period:

denial: "No, this can't be happening to me."
             "It isn't true. It isn't possible."

anger: "How could I be so stupid? I hate myself!"
          "It's all his fault!"
fear: "How can I ever tell my folks?"
          "Will my boyfriend still accept me, or will he leave me?"
          "What will I do about my job? school? college?"
          "What about money?"
          "What will happen to my body?"
          "Having a baby is incredibly painful. I'm afraid!"
panic: "I don't know what to do!"

This is not the time to jump right in with your own agenda for how she should proceed from this point. Instead, listen! Respond to your friend according to *her* needs. This kind of "fellowship" is honoring to God: "Carry each other's burdens, and in this way you will fulfill the law of Christ" (Galatians 6:2).

Get the Facts!

If you're going to share your friend's burden, you have to participate as fully as you can, and part of that participation is knowing all you can know about the dilemma she faces. You may be the only person close to the situation who can keep cool enough to check out the objective facts.

When it comes to pregnancies and unwed parenting, there is a lot to know. So let's start at the beginning.

What is a pregnancy, really?
This question may seem too obvious to ask, but you'd be surprised at how debated it has become in our day.

A pregnancy is *not* just a product of conception, a blob of fetal tissue, or the contents of a uterus. And it's dangerous to use such dehumanizing terminology. A pregnancy is *an unborn child!* And

3

a pregnancy is an unborn child who shares the same basic requirements that all children evidence: food, shelter, and time to grow.

One of many

To you, of course, your friend is not simply a statistic! She is your flesh-and-blood friend with a real-life problem. But it can help to realize that unwed pregnancy is a very widespread problem, and that other girls have faced the crisis and made it!

I learned so much from my entrance into the world of unwed pregnancy. Although I've had older girls stay with me, let's focus on the statistics on teenage pregnancy. More than 1,000,000 teenage girls will become pregnant this year. About 280,000 of these are already married, and another 100,000 will marry after the pregnancy is confirmed. That leaves over 620,000 pregnant, unmarried teens. 400,000 of these pregnancies will be aborted. The remaining 225,000 girls will carry their babies to term. Of this large number, 96 percent will keep their children; that means 210,000 new single mothers each year. Sixty percent of these girls will be pregnant again within two years (*Why Wait*, p. 23).

Eighty percent of pregnant teens drop out of school and never finish. This lack of education is one of the saddest effects of single teenage parenting. It affects the annual income of the young mother for the rest of her life and will also affect the child and his well-being. Seventy percent of unwed teen mothers will go on welfare (*Why Wait*, p. 24). Families headed by young mothers are seven times more likely than other families to be poor. It seems that the key poverty factor for children is whether or not they live in a two-parent family.

Those statistics are so depressing! you're probably thinking. Yes, the figures are grim. And worse yet, these are annual figures! We can't afford to ignore the tough situations our young people face today. Part of the responsibility must be borne by our permissive and increasingly valueless society.

Off to a Good Start

If you've begun by praying for your friend and committing to continue bringing her situation and your friendship before the Lord, if you've communicated—whether verbally or through your supportive actions—that you plan to stick by her during this crisis period, and if you've started to assimilate the information about her situation—you're off to a great start!

Ways to Help

1. Listen and pray!

2. Don't condemn ("Why did you—?" or "How could you—?").

3. Become informed about unexpected pregnancy and the options available to a young woman in your friend's position. Start a file with any information that may be helpful in the future. (See the list of helping agencies in the back of this book. You may want to send for brochures.)

4. Be willing to go with her for a pregnancy test or a doctor's visit.

5. Keep all she has told you confidential, even if others want to talk about the "news" with you.

2

Telling Parents
(and other
significant people)

Maybe you were the first person your friend told about her pregnancy problem. No doubt your friend felt some stress about telling you, even though you are less emotionally connected with the problem than her immediate family or her boyfriend. Consider the importance of her confessions to those important people and their responses to her dilemma.

Some girls tell their boyfriends first. If the "father" reacts negatively, either by denying the problem or by breaking the relationship, your friend will add the pain of his rejection to the emotional whirlwind of her life. If the boyfriend insists on abortion, she has his wishes and that decision to struggle with. Of course, the better informed she is about the development of the baby and the risks of abortion, the harder that decision will be. Ultimately, she risks being abandoned by her boyfriend if she goes against his wishes and chooses life for her child.

Who Needs to Know?

Although there are some young women who become pregnant after they've left their families and are out on their own, most girls facing a problem pregnancy are still dependents in their families. Whether in high school or college, they are not yet ready for independent living.

The parents of these girls should be among the very first to be told. Although parents often turn out to be a pregnant girl's first and best allies, sometimes this can be a difficult hurdle. You can help your friend brave the time of her parents' hurt, disappointment, and anger. Help your friend to realize that, especially if she is still dependent, her parents are her primary emotional and financial resource. No matter what their initial reactions may be, they usually love their daughter very much. Encourage your friend to give her parents time to work through their initial emotional responses. And be especially flexible with your time during this period—she may need it.

Sometimes it is a good idea to have someone help her tell her parents—maybe an older sister, an aunt, a close family relative, a pastor or priest. It is also advisable for your friend to have formulated some tentative plans, some positive options to share with her parents.

Sandy's Story

Sandy felt she would rather run away and disappear into the city than to tell her parents she was carrying a baby. She knew of their high hopes for her and of the special bank account they had established for her college education. How could she hurt them this way?

But somehow Sandy knew that her parents would be more troubled to have her gone completely than to have her with them and troubled. And Sandy had no money and no destination in mind. So there was no way out except to "bite the bullet" and tell them.

She told her mother first. Her mother was very surprised at first, but she seemed calm when she told Sandy, "I'm so sorry this happened—I'm sorry for all of us—but we'll see you through."

She told her dad later that night. He seemed very saddened, but he was loving. They cried together.

Telling them was easier than Sandy had anticipated. And she felt much better knowing that three of them would face the various decisions together.

Sandy has wonderful parents, and many others react with the same love and support they did. But a few parents react quite negatively. Some parents will become angry and hysterical at first, but will be great providers of encouragement, love, and support once they've processed their original hurt and anger. Others from very troubled families will reject their daughters altogether.

Joanne's Story

Some families are so dysfunctional that even slight problems are too great for them to handle. These families can't be counted on for *any* kind of support. A girl from this type of family especially needs a committed-until-the-end friend. Joanne's story is a heartbreaking example of such a home life.

When twenty-year-old Joanne told her parents she was pregnant, her mother and stepfather ordered her to leave by the next day. A day later Joanne found herself without savings, without a job, without a car, and without a place to live. Luckily, she was able to contact a group home and went there to live. In a group home situation, several young women live together with a "houseparent" couple during their pregnancies.

One Tuesday morning my agency called me to ask if I had room for Joanne. "She's been asked to leave the group home immediately. Her baby is due in about sixteen days."

Of course I needed to know why Joanne had to leave the group home. Was it alcoholism, drugs, stealing? Her social worker explained that Joanne had a problem with her attitude toward authority. Joanne's attitude was a bit contagious, and some of the other girls in the home were beginning to rebel as well.

Normally, before a girl comes to live at my house, a preplacement interview is held so that the pregnant young woman can meet me and I can meet her. But because of the emergency of the situation and the fact that the baby was due shortly, I agreed to take her.

So Joanne came. She told me a bit about her family. Her background was rocky, and it was not hard to understand how she had arrived at my door, pregnant and with a poor attitude toward authority figures.

At the time, her mother was going through her fifth divorce. Between marriages, her mother had a succession of live-in boyfriends. Her mother had kicked Joanne out of the house when she was sixteen because Joanne was fighting with her mom's current husband. A year later she came back for a short time but had to leave again under the same circumstances. She'd only been back a second time for a brief period before she was ordered out because of her pregnancy.

In my home, Joanne was feisty and argumentative, but certainly not hostile. Another pregnant girl was also staying with me at the time, and Joanne contradicted almost every statement either of us made. It definitely put a damper on the free flow of conversation around the house. Why speak up if you know before you start that your comments are doomed to be contradicted?

However, we did make some progress in this area. One afternoon when the three of us were in the car heading to a counseling session, I said to her, "Joanne, I get so tired of how you challenge everything I say. Why do you do that?"

She promptly responded with, "I don't challenge everything you say!" Her answer struck the other girl and me as completely funny, and we laughed and laughed. Joanne was a bit put out by our laughter, not understanding that her comment had challenged my remark. But when we explained it to her, she laughed too!

In spite of her problems, Joanne had many good qualities. She loved to cook, was a big help in the kitchen, and enjoyed crafts. She always went to church with me.

But she was either genuinely mistaken or had deliberately not told the truth about her baby's due date, because the sixteen days came and went. Her baby was born after she'd lived with me for two and a half months. Joanne still insists she was pregnant for eleven months!

While staying with me, she became engaged to another young man, not the father of her baby. They planned to marry soon after the baby was born. She asked if she could have an outdoor wedding at my home and wondered if I would help her shop for a dress.

"But Joanne, that's your mother's privilege, and I don't want to take any of it away from her," I protested.

"Oh, my mom would never help me," she replied. "She may not even come to the wedding!"

Poor, bereft Joanne. She had no father, and her mother cared so little for her. Throughout her life Joanne had been searching for crumbs of affection wherever she could find them.

When her little son was born, Joanne released him for adoption and came back to my house to recuperate. A month later her engagement was broken. Now Joanne calls me two or three times a year. Her life-story has grown more complicated. She enlisted in the navy, but was kicked out. She was engaged again, but didn't marry that time either. We've talked about her tendency to head for marriage too quickly. We've talked about her mother's series of husbands and divorces, and I have encouraged her to weigh her decisions more carefully.

Not long ago, Joanne called from another state to tell me she was engaged again and carrying another baby. "I'm going to keep this one!" she exclaimed.

"Does your mother know about your boyfriend and the baby, Joanne?" I asked her.

"My mother moved to Florida and said she never wanted to see me again," she retorted.

Joanne's problems began long before her pregnancy and have continued to follow her. Sadly, many of her inabilities to cope and function successfully in her life are directly connected with the poor parenting she received as a child.

If You Are Mom or Dad

If you are a parent and the pregnant "friend" you are trying to help is your own daughter, realize the importance of the love and support you provide. If there have been difficult patterns of relating established in your home, now is the best time to break them and replace them with a new system of kindness. Ask the Lord to give you patience, wisdom, and a heart full of love for your daughter.

Telling Mom and Dad

It's nearly impossible to predict how your friend's parents will react to her pregnancy. So much depends on the existing dynamics

12

in the family. But their reaction is ultimately critical! Parents' reactions to the pregnancies of their daughters vitally affect the future of those children and grandchildren.

✳ ✳ ✳

Ways to Help

1. Listen and encourage your friend to share with you her fears about telling her parents. Pray through these fears with her.

2. If you know your friend's parents, help her to be realistic about what their responses might be. Maybe you sense that her apprehensions are unreasonable because you know her parents are kind and loving.

3. Go with her to seek counsel from an older person. This may include helping her talk with a pastor or a counselor from a helping agency.

4. Help her come up with some tangible, tentative feelings and plans that she needs to communicate to her parents when she tells them.

5. If needed, offer to go with her when she is going to tell her parents, or give suggestions for someone else who could. Give this careful consideration. Her relationship with her parents may be solid enough for her to tackle the "telling" by herself. If you are not with her, be available for a phone call or a visit immediately after she talks with her parents.

6. Be a good listener and strong support before and after that important interaction with her parents. If her parents make some hurtful remarks during that initial interaction, remind your friend of their hurt and surprise and encourage her to look for some more positive reactions in the days to come.

3

The Unwed Father

It's rather easy to forget about the baby's father—after all, his abdomen is not swelling, his school or career future doesn't seem threatened, etc. But he is a significant piece in the puzzle of your friend's predicament, and your friendship role of support and advice extends to him as well. Most social agencies that work with unmarried pregnant girls are willing and eager to meet with and counsel the unwed father; they are very aware of his importance and of his legal rights and emotional needs.

Maybe the father of the baby is also a friend of yours. Whether or not you have already established a friendship with him, now you can reach out to him by helping him to understand his options and his rights as the baby's father and by meeting some of his needs.

The Hard Truth

The truth of the matter is that most relationships are broken when an unwed pregnancy occurs. In most cases the young men escape the relationship, whether from fear, panic, or disinterest, and the young woman is left to handle the problem by herself. Very few young men remain in contact with the birth mother throughout the entire pregnancy to help her emotionally, and maybe financially, through this difficult time.

Many times a boyfriend will offer to pay for an abortion, and if the pregnant woman refuses, he feels absolved from further responsibility. From my own experience, I have noticed that the young man usually abandons his pregnant partner and has his arms around another girl even before the baby is born.

But before I sound like I have a negative predisposition toward unwed fathers, let me tell you about some of the wonderful ones I have known. Because I am a widow and live alone in a big house in a quiet, unincorporated area, I make it a rule not to take in a girl who is still involved with her boyfriend. This decision was not based on fear, but rather on wisdom, and it makes me and my children feel comfortable. But even I have to bend the rules now and then.

Tough Love

Jim, a seventeen-year-old high school junior, was from out of state. He had permission from his own parents and Peggy's parents to come visit Peggy, who was staying with me during her pregnancy. Peggy's parents called to make arrangements for Jim to spend the weekend at a nearby motel and visit Peggy. By that time Peggy had been with me a month, and I loved and trusted her.

Jim and Peggy had a terrific weekend. They went shopping, to the zoo, and out for pizza. They watched TV together at home. They interacted with me, and I discovered that Jim was a great guy. The more I began to know him, the more I appreciated him. On two subsequent visits, I invited him to stay in my home.

When their baby was born, Jim came to be with Peggy for those three days at the hospital. He demonstrated unusual sensitivity and caring, and Peggy benefited greatly from his emotional support. He was with Peggy in the hospital faithfully, and his tenderness with his baby daughter was touching. With shared tears, they signed the release papers together, knowing that their baby was going to a fine home with parents eager and waiting to love their little girl.

Sharing Peggy's pregnancy experience together and receiving excellent counseling has matured both Peggy and Jim. Great personality growth has resulted. Their tough love for each other and the loving support of both sets of parents made this a truly unusual situation.

Dave's Support

Anne is a delight—a bubbly, happy person, and fun to be with. While staying with me during her pregnancy, she sewed, kept a journal, practiced voice and piano, and worked hard at two college correspondence courses. Dave came from the next state to visit her. I liked him—he was through college and into his first job, and he seemed so right for Anne.

Before discovering Anne's pregnancy, Dave and Anne had set a date, and Anne had picked out a dress. But when they found out Anne had a baby on the way, Dave postponed the wedding.

"I love her so much," he said, "but I'm not ready to be a father!" I had to remind him—though gently—that he already *was* a father.

Anne had already made up her mind that if she and Dave did not marry, she could not keep her baby and parent alone. "But I love him," she said. "And I'll marry him any time he asks me."

"Even if it's after the baby has come and has been placed for adoption?" I asked.

"Even then."

I considered her strong commitment to Dave. I wondered if she and Dave could really get past the difficulties of his decision which allowed her to give their baby away.

When Anne went into labor, she called Dave as she had promised. He arranged to take an entire week off from work, left immediately, and arrived fifteen minutes after his little son was born.

I wondered if seeing that darling boy would inspire Dave to marry Anne right there and then. But that's not how things turned out. Dave spent all of his time with Anne. They cared for their baby, feeding him, singing to him, cradling him, taking pictures of him, and praying over him. And together they cried over the baby as they signed the adoption release papers. Dave stayed at my house during that week, and he was Anne's emotional strength. I was proud of him.

Two weeks later, Anne left just in time to start her spring semester at college. Although quite a distance apart, she and Dave kept in touch with each other by phone, letters, and visits. By midsummer, though, Anne felt the relationship was losing ground and broke it off.

Recently Anne was married to a terrific young man, and I attended their wedding!

Dave and Jim are unusual in that they continued to care and were emotionally involved throughout the whole experience. The result was that both grew in maturity, understanding, and sensitivity.

It's Not Always So Easy

Legally, your friend's partner is called the "putative" father, or alleged father, since your friend could conceivably claim anyone is the father of her child without any proof. Your friend must choose whether or not to name the child's father. And of course, there are legal ramifications which follow her choice.

Naming the Father

If your friend names the father of her baby, the social worker or adviser is usually compelled by law to contact him and advise him of his rights. Legally, he has the right to deny paternity and sign that he is not the baby's father. He can also sign one of two types of surrender—a *surrender for the born child* or a *surrender for the unborn child.*

Sometimes the putative father will not cooperate when the social worker calls him, not responding to letters or not returning any of the necessary forms. In such cases, an attorney representing the agency or the mother eventually will write to the young man to explain his legal options now that he has been named the father of an unborn child. Usually, this contact by an attorney forces the putative father to face his choices and make a decision.

Denying paternity sometimes seems to be the easiest way for a young man to get out of a difficult situation. But usually his denial is emotionally devastating to the baby's mother. She sees her partner walking away from their relationship completely free, while she faces the emotional, financial, and physical stresses of this pregnancy alone. She also faces alone the overwhelming decision of whether to release the child for adoption or parent alone. Signing forms to surrender his parental rights is his other alternative. A father can sign a release of an unborn child before the baby is born, or, like a birth mother, a release for the child a few days after the baby arrives.

In some cases, a putative father may refuse to surrender his rights to the child, declaring that if the mother won't keep the child, he will. Generally, most young women are fairly certain they don't want the father to have sole custody of the baby. So his refusal to surrender becomes a tool for forcing her to keep the baby. Very often, a young father will refuse to sign a surrender until he understands the extent of his own responsibility toward the child if the biological mother keeps the baby.

Recent laws have forced putative fathers seeking paternal rights to be more responsible. Now he must sign a notarized form claiming paternity and stating his desire for paternal rights. Within a set time period, he must appear in court with an attorney to initiate action to establish paternity. This procedure will make him financially responsible for the child and for all the medical bills of the mother. He must also show the presiding judge a childcare plan. If he does not initiate action within the time set by the judge, his rights are automatically terminated.

Not Naming the Father

If your friend chooses not to name the father, another procedure protects his rights. After the child is born, the social worker or legal adviser must advertise for the unknown father living at an unknown address. If he does not come forward within a specific amount of time (approximately thirty days), his rights are terminated.

The choice not to name the father involves some risks. It's not very common, but now and then an "unknown" father *does* turn up within the designated time frame. At this point, the father works through the legal system to determine custody. If a young father seeks custody of his baby, he can be awarded the child if the judge considers him responsible.

In one difficult case a father insisted he wanted to keep the baby, that he had arranged with his mother for the baby's care. But upon investigation, it was discovered that both the young man and his mother were alcoholics, so a petition for unfitness was filed with the court to obtain a release for the baby's adoption.

The young father appeared with an attorney on the first court date and promised to fulfill any requirements to win custody of his child. The judge postponed the hearing for a month. On the second court date, the young man called in, saying that he was having car trouble and couldn't make it. So the judge postponed the hearing again. When the young man did not appear on the third court date, the judge terminated his rights, awarding custody to the adoption agency. But the adoption process had been delayed for five months.

Generally speaking, the arrival of an unnamed father typically puts the whole adoption process into upheaval and often results in a court battle. Most of the time, because the child's biological mother does not want the child to live with his father, the agency returns the child to the unwed mother. After all, they *know* she is the mother; the young man is only an *alleged* father. So a young woman who previously decided that adoption was in the child's best interest may end up keeping her child to prevent her baby from living in a home she considers unsuitable. Sometimes, the putative father's sole reason for seeking custody is to hurt the baby's mother. The pregnancy crisis drags up so many negative emotions and tensions that often their relationship seems poisoned. The unwed father also feels the hurt of that loss.

So the biological mother is thrown back into the turmoil of choosing the best for her baby and often enters into a life of single parenting, and the young father has nothing to show for his attempts to win custody. In most cases, it's best for a girl to name the father so that some of the issues surrounding rights or release can be dealt with before the baby arrives.

If a birth mother chooses to parent her child by herself, the child's named father usually has some visitation rights as well as support responsibilities.

Stay Cool!

Maybe your friend's partner will be a Jim or a Dave and will provide continuing emotional and financial support throughout your friend's crisis experience—I hope so! But if the father of your friend's baby falls into that other 95 percent, stay cool. Your friend will probably feel enough hurt and anger for both of you! You can help her best by listening, praying, and filling part of that support-void she faces. Your added criticisms or "bad-mouthing" won't help her get past the pain. And who knows? Keeping a cool head may even allow you to be able to share information about legal responsibilities with the unwed father.

Ways to Help

1. Help your friend talk about her partner, especially if she is feeling anger and rejection. She will be able to make wiser choices if she has worked through some of these difficult emotions.

2. If you know the father of your friend's baby, encourage him to seek counseling—for himself! If your friend is working with an agency, encourage him to be involved as well. Agencies that

work with unwed mothers also offer services for the birth father.

3. If you are a parent of the unwed father, do not "bad mouth" the unwed young woman. Encourage your son to be as responsible as he can and as involved in the pregnancy as he is permitted to be.

4. If you have negative feelings toward the father of your friend's baby, be careful not to use these feelings to influence your friend.

4

Life or Death?

Once your friend has determined that she is pregnant, she faces a pressing decision about the baby's future. Maybe your friend is convinced that the human life she carries must be given an opportunity to live. Maybe the pressures of her home life, school, work, and friends are making abortion look like a viable option. Especially in the first weeks of panic, an abortion may seem like the ideal solution: "Let's get rid of the problem, and no one ever has to know."

Both you and your friend need to come to terms with the facts about abortion before working toward a decision. The life of an unborn child is not a question to be decided on impulse.

Roe v. Wade

Today abortion has become the hot-button of social issues in America. There are powerful forces at work in our nation on both sides of the question—for and against. Politicians are often elected or rejected on the basis of their position on abortion.

25

The law of our land has made it *legally* acceptable for a mother to decide between life and death for her unborn child (so says the Supreme Court decision of 1973 in the case of Roe v. Wade). You'll notice that I stipulated that this choice is *legally* acceptable; I did not call that choice *morally* acceptable or *physically* acceptable or *emotionally* acceptable. The Roe v. Wade decision of 1973 legalized abortion all across the nation for the entire length of the pregnancy, right up to the day of birth.

But there are many who disagree with this decision. Justice Sandra Day O'Connor has said, "The Roe v. Wade decision is on a collision course with itself." And Justice Harry Blackmun, who wrote the original Roe v. Wade decision, agreed with her: "There is a very distinct possibility that the Court will reconsider Roe v. Wade—maybe even this term" (*Life Docket*, Americans United for Life, October 1988). And he was right. An important case which will require reassessment of Roe v. Wade will soon be addressed by the Supreme Court (*Chicago Tribune,* Jan. 10, 1989).

Because the Roe v. Wade decision leaves two major questions unanswered, it *must* be reviewed. These questions affect people of every age because they deal with human life.

The first question surrounds the organism growing inside a mother: *Is this human life?* (Willke, 1). Exactly what is that growing organism that has the power to change a woman's body chemistry, to affect her moods, to make her sleepy or nauseous? Whatever it is, it's *not dead*. It grows, develops, and replicates its own cells. But is it human life? It has forty-six *human* chromosomes in every cell. It has its own beating heart and circulatory system, separate from the mother's. It's even shaped like a human. And it has its own distinctive set of fingerprints. It doesn't seem to be a bear cub or a potato. It must be, it *is* a human child, needing only time and nourishment and protection to grow, the same needs that all children have.

Roe v. Wade makes abortion legal right up to the day before birth. What is not murder a day before birth becomes murder fifteen minutes after birth. How can we reconcile that fact with logical reasoning or emotions? Our sensibilities rebel against the idea. Awhile ago, newspapers featured the story of a father who threw his newborn son on the floor of the delivery room, killing him. If he had known his child would be born with Down's Syndrome, he would have insisted on abortion. But since he killed his child *after* birth, he was subject to arrest for murder.

That difference of a few hours is horrifying. Of course, the father who killed his son no doubt held unborn human life in low esteem. The jump to just moments after birth was negligible to him.

We must realize that it's a slippery slope from abortion to infanticide to euthanasia (Willke, 245), and that America is sliding down that slope. If life is no longer valuable at its inception, and no longer valuable immediately after birth, the next logical step is the elimination of those who are a costly "burden" to society because they are close to the end of their lives. Strip aside the pretty phrases, "Death with dignity" and "meaningful life," and euthanasia simply means that the doctor has permission to kill the patient. He is, in fact, an accepted murderer.

If his father dies, an unborn child can receive an inheritance on an equal basis with his siblings. Yet his mother can abort him if she chooses. How ironic that we consider him enough of a person to give him money and land, but maybe not life!

If that organism *is* human life, then we must ask the second question: *Should we give equal protection under the law to every human in this nation from the beginning of his life until his death?* (Willke, 2).

There are many cases in lower courts all over the nation that may eventually arrive at the Supreme Court level. Right now there are three cases pending a Supreme Court decision whether to hear the cases or not. One of them, Webster v. Reproductive Health Services, is the case that will soon provide an appropriate opportunity for the Supreme Court to reconsider Roe v. Wade. Another case, Ohio v. Akron Center for Reproductive Health, deals with requiring physicians to notify a minor's parents before performing an abortion—or, if notifying parents is not advisable because of abuse or another reason, to seek permission from a judge.

An organization called *Americans United for Life* is involved with these cases and many others. Comprised of pro-life attorneys dedicated to re-establishing legal protection of our nation's unborn children, the organization brings cases to trial, defends others, and drafts model legislation to chip away at the edges of the Roe v. Wade-related court decisions.

Think About It

Many times this awesome decision of life or death is thrust upon a young person who does not yet understand all the ramifications of the decision she has to make. Often she does not know that even before she is sure she is pregnant the baby's heart is beating—it begins twenty-four days after conception. At thirty days, his own blood—separate from the mother's—is flowing in his veins.

Believe it or not, a girl younger than eighteen does not have to have her parents' permission to get an abortion. Of course, she can't get her ears pierced without their written permission, but she can have abortive surgery! Most of the time, a girl this young does not want to tell her parents, so she and her boyfriend scrape together the fees for the abortion, or she withdraws money from her own savings. Then this young girl, quietly and secretly, undergoes a major surgical procedure on her body.

Although this fourteen-, fifteen-, sixteen-, seventeen-year-old teenager cannot legally sign a contract, hold a title to real estate, or perhaps even drive a car, she can legally sign a document at an abortion clinic that absolves the clinic and its doctors from any responsibility if there are medical complications. The following is part of the document from a California abortion clinic.

> I know that the practice of medicine and surgery is not an exact science and that reputable practitioners cannot properly guarantee results. I acknowledge that no guarantee or assurances have been made by anyone regarding the operation which I have requested and authorized. I understand that certain unfavorable results may follow the operation, including, but not limited to, pain and suffering, bleeding, sterility, and emotional upset (Baker, 23).

The clinic admits that serious complications may occur. Does such a young girl even know what *sterility* means or understand how it might affect her future happiness? How twisted the thinking of our society can be—when a young person who cannot have her ears pierced without adult supervision can sign a form like this one without her parents' knowledge!

This process is hardly fair to a girl's parents, either. If "certain unfavorable results" do occur, the parents will be the ones to carry the responsibility of picking up the pieces and paying any medical costs. And if their daughter never shares her secret with them, they may not even be aware of her emotional needs and scars.

Believe It or Not

In one case, *Americans United for Life* represented a mother who was deliberately deceived by a junior-high teacher to prevent her knowledge about or interference with her daughter's abortion (Condon, 10-11). In the case of Preston v. Thermalito School District, the teacher made arrangements for the abortion and for state funding to cover the cost. The teacher also wrote a note to the young girl's mother, explaining that the daughter was going to babysit over the weekend when actually the girl was going to have an abortion.

The first Mrs. Preston knew about her daughter's abortion was when someone called from an emergency room where her daughter was being treated for complications. What a nightmare for that family!

The teacher, the principal, the School Board, the School District, the School Superintendent, the doctor who performed the abortion, and the clinic where it took place were all named defendants in the lawsuit. This case was settled out of court before it reached trial, with all except the School Superintendent participating in the settlement; he is still under consideration.

That case provides a good illustration of how Roe v. Wade is damaging to our society. It demonstrates that the law of the land can undermine the strength of the family structure. A school nurse can't give a thirteen-year-old an aspirin without checking with her parents, but a teacher can take the same young girl for an abortion, an abortion paid for by the state. What kind of logic is being employed in such a decision?

It gets worse: When complications—physical or emotional— arise, who is responsible to pick up the pieces and live with the damage inflicted by a procedure which took place outside their knowledge or consent? The parents—not the state. Reread that disclaimer from an abortion clinic. Possible complications include pain and suffering, bleeding, sterility, and emotional upset. The unborn child is not the only victim of an abortion; so is the young girl. And perhaps she is the more tragic victim.

Sooner or later, our country will decide about abortion at the level where it began: the Supreme Court. This is not the first time in our nation's history that the highest court made a bad decision. The Supreme Court's Dred Scott decision of 1857 determined that a black slave had no rights as a person but was merely property, subject to the decisions of his owner. An owner even could choose life or death for that slave. That was three years before Abraham Lincoln became President; the decision was reversed after the Civil War because it failed to provide equal protection for all men. In a similar way, Roe v. Wade stripped the unborn child of "equal protection under the law."

What About Extreme Cases?

People often argue for abortion on the basis of the extreme and unusual cases. An example would be when the pregnant mother of four young children is likely to die in childbirth if she carries the fifth child to term. First of all, these cases are extremely rare. So rare, in fact, that in all my reading, I have never come across such a case.

Carrying a baby as the result of rape or incest is another extreme case. Together these two extreme cases—rape and incest—constitute only 1 percent of the abortions done each year. The other 99 percent of abortions are sought for personal, social, and economic reasons (Willke, 151).

I had mixed feelings myself about abortion after rape—until I met Beth.

God at Work

Beautiful, blonde Beth was the daughter of missionaries to South America. She was eighteen, had just graduated from high school, and was looking forward to college and a career in nursing.

Beth was the victim of rape. She had attended a party at a girlfriend's house, a home she had often visited before. She went upstairs to leave her coat on one of the beds. As she stepped into a

31

darkened bedroom, the door was closed and locked behind her. A young man wrestled her to the bed and sexually assaulted her.

By the time Beth finished her story, we were both crying. "Oh, Beth—how horrible!" I exclaimed. "Didn't you kick or bite or scream or scratch?"

"I was afraid to; I didn't dare. I didn't know who he was. He was stronger—I was afraid he was on drugs or drunk; I thought he was going to kill me. But I prayed! I prayed, 'Please, Lord, don't let me get pregnant.' "

Beth didn't know that medical help was available after a rape, and she did not tell her parents about it. She hid in her room, pretending to be sick; she was physically and emotionally traumatized.

Eventually she discovered that she was pregnant, and she was devastated. She told her parents the whole story; her father was concerned about her and furious toward the young man. He tried to trace the young man through friends who had been at the party, only to discover that he had moved to another city right after the rape.

Beth's parents knew nothing about helping agencies in the United States. They felt they had to resign from the mission and come back to the United States to see their daughter through her pregnancy. Beth was firmly against the idea of abortion. "This baby is half mine," she said. "I don't know why I am pregnant—I asked God to protect me from it. But I can't destroy the baby." Beth's difficult decision is quite mature, considering her age and that she was a victim of rape.

Beth's dad called the director of their mission board to tell him about the problem and offer their resignation. The mission director immediately told them about the agency I work with, an agency that would care for Beth throughout the pregnancy and delivery and would handle an adoption to a two-parent Christian home. When Beth's father heard that Beth would live in a caring foster home at no cost to their family, he decided to look into the option. He called the agency all the way from South America to hear about the program first-hand. He was completely convinced that this would be a wise way to go.

But Beth's mom had doubts about sending her daughter far away to total strangers during such a difficult time. So Beth and her mom came together from South America to check things out. I met their plane and took them home to stay as long as they wanted.

Since I had reservations for a Living Bibles Banquet that night, we went together. We were seated at a table with Dr. Ken Taylor, the translator of the *Living Bible*. It was God's miraculous provision. Later I discovered that Beth's family was using the English translation in their home but did not have access to the Spanish Living Bible. Beth's mom knew it would be a useful tool for teaching her Spanish women's Bible class.

So after spending time in my home and interviewing with the agency, Beth's mom went back to South America with her questions answered and her doubts resolved—carrying two dozen Spanish *Living Bibles*!

Five months later, Beth delivered a lovely baby girl. She had long before decided that she would not keep this baby that resulted from such a brutal, traumatic experience, but she spent a great deal of time with her daughter in the hospital. When I came to pick her up, the baby was with her in her room. We took pictures, and Beth said her final good-byes, and we wheeled the little cart back to the nursery. Beth was weeping, and my heart ached for her. The whole experience was a very difficult time in her life, and I greatly admired her courage.

Before knowing Beth, I had been ambivalent regarding the question of abortion after a rape. Of course my sympathies were always with the girl who had experienced such violence. It seemed almost unreasonable to "punish" her further by making her carry a rapist's baby to term.

But living with Beth forced me to think more deeply about this whole issue of rape and abortion. Yes, rape is a violent act against a young woman's body. But abortion is also a violent act against the same body. A second violent act cannot cancel out the first; the memory and trauma of the rape would remain, compounded by the eventual realization that she had ended a baby's life.

Seeing that beautiful, perfect little girl in Beth's arms made me realize that no matter how that baby was conceived, she did not deserve to be killed. Why should there be *two* victims to a rape?

I learned so much from Beth. It takes a mature and unselfish girl to carry a rape baby to term. Beth believed in the value of that human life—in spite of the painful memories the pregnancy brought—enough to give that baby the gift of life.

Ways to Help

1. Spend time with your friend investigating the development of an unborn baby: at what week the heart beats, when the fingers and toes are distinct, etc.

2. Educate yourself about abortion and the pro-life movement, and pray about how you can help preserve the value of human life.

3. Find out and provide the phone numbers for the resources available to your friend.

5

Facts About Abortion: How It's Done

Abortion—the term is abstract, distant, a word people can hear without discomfort. But the real thing is a whole new ballgame—it's the destruction of beating hearts, tiny fingers and toes, actual arms and legs. Before we even begin, I'll tell you that it is an ugly subject.

Let's take a look at several methods of abortion.

How It's Done

Suction

The suction method is commonly used early in the pregnancy. The abortionist stretches the cervix (opening to the womb) to insert a suction instrument into the uterus. This mechanism is a hollow, plastic tube with a sharp, knife-like edge at the tip. The suction tears the baby's body into pieces. The abortionist then cuts the placenta from the inner wall of the uterus. All the parts are sucked out by the tube into a bottle. Legs, arms, head, and hips are often easily recognizable (Willke, 86).

D and C

The D and C (dilation and curettage) method does not employ suction. Instead, the abortionist inserts a curette (a loop-shaped, steel knife) into the uterus. He cuts the baby and the placenta into pieces and scrapes them out into a basin.

D and E

The D and E (dilation and evacuation) method is used after the unborn child is twelve weeks old. A pliers-like instrument is needed at this point because the baby's bones (especially the skull) are calcified. The unborn child is not anesthetized. The abortionist inserts the instrument into the uterus, seizes a leg or other part of the body and tears it with a twisting motion from the baby's body. The action is repeated again and again, snapping the spine, crushing the skull. A nurse stands by to reassemble the small, broken body to ensure that all the body parts have been removed from the mother's womb.

Saline poisoning

Salt poisoning (saline amniocentesis) is done after the baby is sixteen weeks old. A large needle is inserted through the mother's abdominal wall and into the baby's amniotic sac. A concentrated salt solution is injected into the amniotic fluid. The baby swallows the poison as he breathes, struggles, and sometimes convulses. It takes over an hour to kill the baby. When the process is successful, the mother goes into labor approximately twenty-four hours later and delivers a dead baby (Willke, 86). The outer layer of the baby's skin is often burned away by the salt solution. When the dead child is delivered, he often looks raw and red.

Abortion pills

The Upjohn company is the first major drug company to switch from producing only drugs that will save lives and alleviate suffering to producing a drug that kills. They have begun marketing a hormonal drug that induces abortions. For this reason, many pro-life people have stopped using Upjohn products (Willke, 87). Upjohn has withdrawn one of its abortion-inducing products from the marketplace in response to public pressure. (For more information about Upjohn products and a list of equivalent alternative brands, contact the *Right to Life of Cincinnati* at the address listed in the resource section at the back of this book.)

Hysterotomy

When a pregnancy is well advanced, the method of hysterotomy is sometimes employed. Hysterotomy is the medical term for an early Caesarean section. This method involves major surgery. The mother's abdomen and uterus are cut, and the baby is lifted out. If the baby is strong enough to breathe and survive, it is often smothered, starved, plunged into a bucket of water, or put to death by some other barbaric practice. A live birth from an abortion is considered a "medical complication." At this point we've crossed over from killing babies in the womb to killing them after they are born. I call that *infanticide*, not abortion.

Megan's Choice

Megan is a tiny girl. She still looks seventeen, although she's well into her twenties now. She has a loving husband and three beautiful children, but the evidences of her deep grief reveal themselves in her eyes when she talks about the child she doesn't have.

Megan's Christian family was a quiet one, and they had a hard time demonstrating their love to one another. Megan herself was shy, and didn't develop the normal close friendships with other girls. She started dating Curt during her junior year of high school. His affectionate ways and his large, loving family warmed Megan's heart, and she began to feel good about herself and to lose some of her withdrawn ways. Curt and Megan knew pretty quickly that they loved each other, and they dreamed about their future together. When Megan was a senior in high school, she and Curt slept together, and Megan became pregnant.

Megan and Curt made plans to marry after graduation, but when they told Megan's parents, her folks were furious and ashamed. They insisted on abortion as the solution to the problem. Megan had always obeyed her parents and was even afraid of her father; so, although she and Curt fought the decision, she eventually had an abortion—paid for by Megan's parents.

Megan enrolled at the Christian college her parents chose for her, but she continued to see Curt every weekend. She dropped a great deal of weight, remained aloof from college life, did poorly in her classes (although she had been a good student in high school), and cried in her sleep. Her roommates and school counselor became concerned and began asking questions, but her parents warned her not to tell anyone.

Megan suffered her grief for her unborn child alone. Not even Curt could feel that same pain. She, like many other women who have had abortions, experienced overwhelming sadness and guilt.

After resolving some of the hurts in her family and finding comfort in the love of Christ, she and Curt eventually married, and they have a growing family. "I know I'm forgiven, and I think I even forgive myself now," she says, "but both Curt and I know our baby was a *real child*. I thought having children would ease the sense of loss I feel. I love my children so much, and I find so much joy in parenting them, but I can't forget my unborn baby."

So Many Others

More and more women are discussing the personal problems that follow an abortion. They describe emotional reactions: "guilt, anger, depression, fear of discovery, loss of ability to experience emotions, and painful reactions when encountering pregnant women or small children" ("Women of Abortion Speak Out," *Christianity Today*, 11/18/88). Others experience lingering problems such as extreme weight gain or loss (like Megan), drug or alcohol abuse and addiction, promiscuity, repeat pregnancies, flashbacks, and nightmares ("Women of Abortion Speak Out").

And almost all of them change their minds about abortion. After the abortion, approximately 96 percent of the women regarded abortion as wrong ("Women of Abortion Speak Out").

The Inside Story

Many times a pregnant girl considers her own feelings and life situation but neglects to think about the growing life in her womb. The following acrostic, written by a sensitive seventh-grade girl, shares the inside perspective—from the view of the baby.

The Inside Story

A s a growing feeling of excitement
B uilds up inside of me, the passing of time becomes endlessly slow.
C osily snuggled within the warm body of my mother, I
D ream of what I am and will become in my promising future.
E very thought that passes through my mind is
F earless and secure, but the
G race my life is filled with will soon pass.
H appy birthday!" I say to myself, for today

I am six months old. Yet even when I am
J oyful I
K now something is wrong.
L ater in the day I feel a prodding on my back,
and I wonder if it's my
M other. Somehow though, I sense that it is someone else,
and I am
N ervous.
O utside of me loud voices fill the room.
I know they are talking about me, but I am
P uzzled as to what they are saying,
for I trust them too completely to suspect any danger.
Q uickly though it comes to me.
These people that were meant to
R aise me, or at least love me, are plotting my murder.
S ilently with little nudges and quiet phrases
I plead with my mother.
T hey are planning an abortion and saying it is only between
the doctor and the patient, but they do not
U nderstand that they are leaving someone
V ery important out. Me!
W eeping softly, sobs shake my mother as the doctor
X -rays her thin frame.
Y oung and naive as she is, my mother doesn't realize or even
suspect that on next Tuesday when I am torn from her,
it will create a wound that even time will not heal.
Z ealous for her own life she's neglecting mine.

Kari Cade

The poet used her imagination to realize that an unborn child is *a person*. Her insight is invaluable. Who knows what creativity and greatness lie in the wombs that are being emptied today?

Mary's Choice

Seventeen-year-old Mary discovered that she was pregnant. Thankfully, she had a good relationship with her parents, and she was able to tell them about it.

"Of course you will get an abortion," her mother said, as if the matter were settled.

"No, Mom," replied Mary, "I've thought about it a lot. I don't want to destroy my baby. I want to keep the child."

"But, Mary—you can't! You'll ruin your life. We simply won't let you." Mary's mom's face had taken on a strained and panicked look.

"Your mother is right," Dad joined in. "You have so much potential. I want to see you go to college."

What Mary's parents didn't know was that Mary had already experienced abortion. She'd had one secretly the year before. She'd read a lot about abortion since then, and she had never stopped feeling terrible inside about the death of that first baby. No wonder she was so positive she didn't want another abortion!

But because they weren't aware of Mary's earlier trauma, her parents continued to pressure her until the tension at home got so bad that Mary went to stay with her married brother. There she learned about an agency that could help her.

The agency found her a home with a helpful, caring couple who had two preschool-aged children and another pregnant girl living with them. There Mary received excellent counseling week after week, helped with the children, read extensively, and waited for her baby in a peaceful, supportive, loving atmosphere. Those months of observing the day-to-day care of young children and the enormous, long-term responsibilities of parenting affected her deeply. She realized that parenting was quite a challenge even in a two-parent home, and she knew that she was not yet ready to parent her baby alone.

41

Her parents were right; Mary did have a great deal of potential. She wanted to go to college as much as her parents wanted her to go. And her decision to give her baby life and then to release him for adoption would allow her to achieve that goal of education and maturity. It took more time and consideration and love to follow through on that decision, but Mary felt at peace about it in her heart.

Choose Life!

Your friend carries within her a life—a *human* life—that is entitled to "equal protection" whether the government says so or not. Your friend is the baby's primary guardian and protector. Help her face the facts about abortion and do what you can to help her choose life!

Once your friend has made the momentous decision—the decision to give life to the child—other decisions will follow. The baby is going to live, but how will the mother live during and after the pregnancy? What about school or work? What about parenting or adoption? In the next chapters, we'll tackle those questions one at a time.

✳ ✳ ✳

Ways to Help

1. Familiarize yourself with information on the methods and risks of abortion, and help your friend understand some facts.

2. Discuss with your friend how she feels about the baby. Is she angry? fearful? resentful? Gently remind her that her baby is

her *baby*—not an "it." Help her to think through the whole situation clearly.

3. Pray for your friend as she makes this decision. It will affect both her future and that of her baby.

6

To Parent or Not to Parent

When a young woman has chosen to give life to her child, usually her initial plan is to parent the child. This is a natural and normal response. A woman was created to cuddle and cradle that newborn who was nurtured in her womb for nine months.

But there is much more to parenting than simple cuddling. It is advisable for your friend to receive counseling early in the pregnancy, preferably from a skilled social worker or counselor. The counselor will help your friend to assess her readiness to parent and to consider every advantage and disadvantage regarding both parenting and releasing for adoption. A wise counselor can help her weigh the pros and cons of parenting, and can describe the immense changes that a baby will make in her life and future. Both parenting and releasing a baby for adoption can be positive experiences and a means of growth and maturing for your friend.

Whatever your friend decides, things will never be the same; she will always have either the child or the memory of her child.

A young woman may change her mind about what to do many times throughout her pregnancy. Don't worry if your friend keeps changing her mind. It means she is working through the decision, thinking deeply about it. A child's future is a decision worth taking time for!

Some Things to Consider

A baby is a miracle. If your friend chooses to parent, she will enjoy her child's presence and personality and growth—the first smile, the first tooth, the first word, the first wobbly steps. All parents delight in these elements of parenting! But the delights balance out against the responsibilities: the insistent presence of the child, the almost constant feeding initially, keeping that baby clean, the expense, and the sleepless nights.

In those first miracle moments in the hospital, it's hard to consider that a baby is a long-term commitment—a life-time! But your friend needs to consider the impact of her baby's arrival on her personal future. If your friend chooses to parent, her freedom to come and go as she pleases will be severely curtailed. Her social life as a single mother will be limited.

A young single mother often faces a difficult financial situation. If she has not completed her schooling and has no job experience, she will struggle to find employment which pays much more than minimum wage. Such a salary cannot maintain an apartment and a car, pay for child care, and feed both mother and baby. It is very difficult for a young mother to remain in good spirits and emotional health when the lack of financial stability continually gnaws at her.

If all else fails, a young mother is often forced to go on Public Aid. Although at first this appears to be a good solution, it usually becomes a dead-end street. The dependency is damaging to the young woman's self-esteem and often stifles personal ambition. And sadly, this welfare mentality often transfers to the next generation. Many people remain on Public Aid, even to a second or third generation.

Finances are a crucial area for any family. Anticipating the needs of your friend will enable her to meet them better. Use the ideas listed below to help your friend get a clear perception of the money she will need to care for herself and her baby.

Starter Expenses

Some items are necessities in preparing to be a parent. Your friend will need to rent a furnished place or furnish an apartment herself. Find out what furnished places cost to rent. Add up the costs of a bed, a dresser, a sofa, chairs, a table, etc. Use catalogs, classified ads in papers, or go window-shopping to determine the prices of these items. You might also check Salvation Army and Good Will resale shops.

Household items add up, too. What about dishes, pots and pans, utensils, towels, and sheets?

And the baby will have some special needs. Find out what baby furniture costs: bassinets, a crib, a dresser or changing table, baby bathtub, car seat, playpen. What about a layette for the baby? The child will require diapers, undershirts, sleepers, socks, and some outfits. Call someone who has a new baby and ask how many of each item you will actually need (how many diapers each week, how many outfits). And baby magazines in the doctor's waiting room sometimes feature a list of necessary items.

Surprisingly, keeping a baby seems to cost as much as keeping an adult! Your friend should also estimate the more everyday costs of towels and cloths, formula, baby oil and baby powder, bottles, nipples, sterilizers, baby vitamins, and baby food.

If your friend plans to parent her baby, you might want to help her by planning a baby shower. Depending on the circumstances, this can be a great, practical way to get her started.

Month-to Month Expenses

Your friend should try to guess/estimate her monthly income. If she doesn't have a job now, call the state employment office and check the classified ads. Help her evaluate her education and skills to determine an attainable salary level.

Once you've got some idea of what her cash flow might be like, help her anticipate what the monthly expenses of living on her own with the baby will entail.

Rent, of course, is the first consideration. Call a real estate agent for information, or search the classified ads for ideas. Don't forget your list of costs for household furnishings. Would it be less expensive for your friend to rent a furnished place or to furnish a place by herself? How does she feel about having a one-bedroom place? Can she afford a two-bedroom?

Utilities add up. Call a few apartment complexes to ask about the average cost of utilities each month. Call the phone company and ask them about costs for installation and about monthly local and long-distance rates.

If your friend plans to work and care for her baby, she will most likely need a car. If she has one already, add up her monthly payment, her monthly insurance payment, and estimate monthly costs of gas and maintenance. If your friend is planning to do her best without a car, using public transportation, help her estimate how many trips she'll take each month, including trips to the doctor, to the grocery store, or to visit friends and grandparents. How much do these trips add up to?

As a single parent, your friend will probably have to work. Find out the hourly rates for babysitting in the area where she lives. About how many hours will your friend need a paid babysitter each week? Check out the local daycare centers to find out their monthly rates. Sometimes these costs are kept down because a willing relative offers to look after the baby.

Medical costs are especially important. Call your friend's doctor's office to discuss the routine exams required for a baby and a new mother. Ask about costs. Try to find out if there are clinics in your friend's area that have sliding-scale fees (payments based on income). If your friend already has insurance, call her company to determine monthly costs of insurance coverage.

Help your friend plan a week of meals for herself and the baby. Then make up a grocery list for that week. Have some fun in the grocery store, shopping without buying! Add up the costs of the items on the list and multiply that week by four or five to estimate monthly food costs. Ask a friend who is an experienced shopper if your estimate is accurate.

Help your friend assess what she typically spends in a month on personal needs such as haircuts, clothes, toiletries, and entertainment. Help her come up with ideas for cutting those costs down a little. Come up with a tentative monthly amount (this area is one of the more difficult to estimate in advance). Add up the various monthly amounts—for rent, utilities and phone, transportation, babysitting and medical costs. Do the monthly costs come within the range of your friend's monthly income?

All in the Family

Surely one advantage of parenting as an option is that the child will be with his biological parent. He will also be a part of his mother's natural background, with his natural grandparents and other family members. He might have Cousin Albert's nose or Aunt Ramona's red hair.

There are flip sides to these advantages, though. Those family members might have rejected the young mother, creating an atmosphere of tension and disharmony or leaving her alone with her responsibility altogether. The baby's biological mother will likely have to work to provide for the two of them. Full-time employment, errands, and other activities (like further education or church-related events) will leave that baby in the care of other people for forty to fifty hours *minimum* each week. This constant separation could lead to feelings of insecurity or frustration—on the parts of both mother and child. Sometimes it means less than adequate training and discipline in those early formative years, depending on the skill and love of the caretaker.

The baby's being with his biological mother also most often means life without a father figure in the home. Many people mistakenly assume that a father figure is more important for a young boy, but it is equally important for the development of a girl. A baby was meant to have both mother and father. Temporary father figures may or may not help. Sometimes they simply lead to further insecurity in a child.

There is also the possibility of a stepfather someday. This solution is wonderful when a man bonds to and loves his wife's child as his own, which often happens. But the child's insecurity problem is in a precarious position if the new father is distant or abusive.

Of course the day-to-day and financial responsibilities are eased when there is a father to share the burdens. But help your friend see the danger of jumping prematurely into marriage, hoping to ease the financial strain. Statistics show that 90 percent of teen marriages made because of a pregnancy fail within six years.

Molly and Joe make a great example of two teens who married, only to find that the financial situation didn't get any easier.

Molly

As a sixteen-year-old sophomore, Molly lived with her divorced father and his second wife. She was a tiny teen, weighing scarcely more than a hundred pounds, but she was "full of vinegar." Constantly at war with her dad, she hated school, and had already run away from home twice.

The only place she found affirmation was with Joe, a seventeen-year-old friend. They became sexually involved. When she became pregnant, she knew her father would react badly, so she ran away. There was no girlfriend that she could call, no other family to whom she could go. So she slept in a small local park for three nights and wandered in town during the days. She never went back to school.

But Joe knew where she was. In desperation he went to the police and asked what would happen if Molly turned herself in. The police told him that one of two agencies in town would give her shelter. Joe and Molly finally went to the police station to seek a solution to their dilemma. A local youth outreach organization in the business of helping runaway teens sent one of their staff to pick up Molly. She came to stay with me, temporarily.

She arrived with nothing but the clothes on her back and Joe's sweater—not even a toothbrush or hairbrush. What little money she'd had was spent on food during those three days of wandering. I quickly went out to get her some personal items.

Because Molly was three months pregnant, she was put in the care of another agency. That agency placed her in a loving foster home that was already housing two other very young pregnant teens. She stayed there in a peaceful, accepting, happy household

51

through the rest of her pregnancy. She received good counseling from the agency in the decisions she was facing. And Molly came to know Christ as her Savior during that time.

Molly and Joe wanted to marry. However, in retaliation for all the aggravation she had caused him, her father refused to sign for her. Her mother lived somewhere in the south, and Molly had long ago lost touch with her.

Molly eventually delivered a healthy little boy and decided to keep her baby, although she had no home, no job, no family to help, and Joe was still a high-school junior. Her plans for the future were contained in the phrase, "Something will turn up—it always does." As a last resort, Joe's mother took her in. There were already five younger brothers and sisters living in that home, and the family was on Public Aid.

Joe and Molly lived there as a married couple while she took care of the child and Joe stayed in school, working at part-time jobs as much as he could. By the time he graduated, they had a second son. A month after the arrival of baby number two, Molly turned eighteen, and she and Joe were married. Joe had hoped to become a broadcaster, but with a wife and two sons to support, there is little chance he will be able to pursue further schooling.

Molly and Joe are working hard to make their marriage work. I pray that they do, although the future looks pretty bleak. Joe and Molly are still on Public Aid, just as Joe's parents are.

"I'm Ready"

When Lois was thirty years old, she went through a divorce after six years of marriage. She and her husband had no children, although she had wanted them. During her marriage she and her husband had not used birth control, and she had never become pregnant. The doctors had been unable to pinpoint the problem.

When her husband discovered that he loved someone else and wanted to divorce Lois, Lois didn't seem to have much choice. She agreed, and they separated.

Even before her divorce became final, Lois became involved with another man and soon found that she was pregnant. She was astounded and very happy, because she had believed that she was sterile.

Lois never questioned whether she should carry the baby to term. After receiving wise counseling, she decided, "I'm ready to parent!" Her good job was secure, her income stable, and her home situation roomy enough to add a child. She felt ready and eager to take on the responsibility. She felt glad, too, that because she had been married and very recently divorced, no stigma of illegitimacy would attach itself to her baby. Her family was positive about her choice. She happily accepted the parenting of her son, and today they are doing well.

Not Quite All Alone

When a young woman remains at home with her baby, her child is often reared mainly by the grandparents. This generally works very well because it allows the young woman stability for the year or two it takes for her to finish school or become established on her own. Many grandparents take great delight in helping to nurture their daughter's child. But sometimes grandparents feel it is their "duty" to help parent their child's child, while inwardly resenting the great changes the new responsibility has made in their personal lives.

Other times a set of grandparents will adopt their grandchild. This is one solution, but of course there are possible difficulties. In the case of Norene's family, what started out as "the best for all concerned" didn't turn out so well.

Norene had her baby daughter when she was sixteen. She stayed at home with her parents, and all agreed that the best possible solution was for Norene's parents to adopt little Joanne. So Norene's parents adopted their granddaughter, and Norene was able to finish high school and get a good job. At no time did she provide the primary care or any financial help for Joanne, and there was really no reason that she should have. Her daughter had become her "little sister" legally. Of course, she loved Joanne very dearly and felt like Joanne's mother in her heart, but Joanne called her grandmother "Mommy."

When Norene was twenty, she chose to marry and wanted to take her daughter/sister with her. Joanne, at four, looked exactly like her biological mother. She was beautiful, and it pleased Norene very much.

"No way," said Norene's mother. "Joanne belongs to us, and she stays here! It can't be good for her to disrupt the family she's known and understood."

There were long and bitter fights between Norene and her parents. No doubt Joanne was confused about why her "Mommy" and her sister were fighting about her.

Finally, Norene and her boyfriend simply went to the Justice of the Peace to get married. They didn't even have a wedding celebration. Today, Norene and her mother never speak to one another and never see each other, and Joanne is growing up in the home of her grandparents (legally, her parents).

The family decision seemed like a good solution at first, but four years later it split that family apart.

A Story of Struggle and Success

While many parents are very eager to offer financial and supportive help if their daughter chooses to parent her child, a few react quite negatively. Lorraine's case was an especially painful one, considering the extreme disruption of her family that resulted from her crisis.

Lorraine was a pretty, twenty-six-year-old brunette who came to live with me three days before Christmas one year. She had never lived away from home before. She was six and a half months pregnant. Her parents were having a Christmas party and didn't want their relatives to see that Lorraine was pregnant, so they decided it was time for Lorraine to come to my house.

Lorraine's parents had emigrated from eastern Europe, and the forceful father ruled his home with an iron fist. Lorraine's dilemma triggered a constant stream of anger and verbal abuse from her father. She was "no good" and a "disgrace to the family."

Lorraine was a bright girl with a good job—she had worked at one large firm for eight years. Her car was her own and completely paid for. She also had a healthy savings account. So, despite her father's angry threats, she determined to keep her baby.

Although her father called weekly to insist she give up the baby for adoption and to threaten Lorraine and her unborn child, she pursued her parenting plan responsibly and enthusiastically. Week after week she scanned the housing section of the newspaper for an apartment to rent, and two weeks before she had the baby she found one—just a few miles from her office. She continued to work until the day before the birth and spent her free hours furnishing her little home with the bare necessities.

Her father's irate phone calls continued. "You will never darken my door again! I'll forget I ever had a daughter such as you! I will never call that kid my grandchild! If I ever see you with that kid in your arms, I'll grab it and bash its head on the sidewalk!" His anger was only compounded by the frustrating fact that his threats seemed to have no effect on his daughter; she was sure she wanted to keep her baby.

When he phoned me, he encouraged me to break her confidence. He insisted that I tell her to "give up" her baby and that she could never be a "fit" mother.

I was definitely camping on Lorraine's side against this unreasonable, malignant anger. I responded calmly, "It's Lorraine's baby and Lorraine's future. Only she can make a decision about the baby—"

He screamed at me, accusing me of being a "religious person" who stuck my nose into other people's business! Since there was no dealing with him, I did the best thing possible—hang up.

Lorraine bravely and beautifully delivered a baby girl. As she lay with the baby in her arms in the delivery room, Lorraine looked at me with tears, saying, "He can't make me give her up, can he?"

"No, dear," I reassured her. "She's yours, and the decision belongs to you."

Lorraine called her mother that morning to tell her the news. Later the same day her father called the hospital to repeat his threats and insults. Lorraine was upset by the call and talked with me again about her father's anger. She didn't want his disappointment and anger to influence her decision about the baby. Finally I left her and went home.

I was barely in the door when my phone rang. Lorraine was sobbing. She had just endured a second abusive call from her father and was too distressed to relax. "Why don't we have the hospital switchboard deny your incoming calls, Lorraine?" I suggested. She agreed, and I made the arrangement.

Somehow her father's call still got through the next afternoon. Lorraine was so upset by the call that I took the phone from her and put it to my ear.

I identified myself and asked, "Sir, are you *never* going to forgive your daughter?"

"Never! She is as good as dead to me."

"I understand your anger," I said, "but haven't *you* ever done anything wrong in your lifetime?"

"That has nothing to do with it!" He was furious.

"Sir," I said, "Lorraine tells me that you believe in God. God says we have to forgive others just the way we expect God to forgive us—"

"Enough!" he shouted, and he slammed down the phone.

The poor new mother was exhausted, and I spoke to the head nurse again about denying Lorraine's calls.

The next day, I took Lorraine and her daughter to their new apartment. In the days that followed, I visited them with some hot meals. Their new life together had begun. Six weeks later I attended the baby's christening ceremony at a local church; although Lorraine's mother was present and supportive, her father was not there.

After a six-week maternity leave, Lorraine went back to her good-paying job, and the lovely little girl went to a good babysitter. I saw the little family on the baby's first birthday, and daughter and single mom were doing well.

Life's an Adventure

One of the girls who stayed with me discovered that "life's an adventure." She was ready to accept the challenge of parenting by the time her baby arrived.

They say there's a calm within every storm. During my second pregnancy as an unwed mother, I found that calm in a friendship filled with understanding, acceptance, and support.

When I was nineteen, I placed a beautiful, healthy daughter for adoption. Although I dearly loved my little girl and felt good about my decision of adoption, I was not prepared for the grief, confusion, and anger that followed our separation. I found myself back in the same relationship, and three years later I was pregnant again.

My life was pretty much a mess. I couldn't accept abortion as an alternative, but I couldn't accept my pregnancy. My mother was terrific and would have permitted me to stay at home, but I couldn't face other people because I didn't have any answers to the questions they presented. I worried about my two young nephews, who are very dear to me. I didn't want them to think that sex and bringing a baby into the world were things to be taken lightly.

Staying at Henrietta's gave me time to deal with my pregnancy and my changing appearance, and it gave my family time to sort out their feelings. Henrietta provided helpful acceptance and objectivity. She made it clear by her actions and attitudes that she was a friend, not a "surrogate mother." I was permitted to go through different, necessary stages. I cried the tears, was scared, struggled with the reality, discovered the love for my baby, was angry and weak, found forgiveness and strength, and made decisions—all without judgments or advice and opinions that I didn't ask for. There were days when I wanted to have someone tell me what to do, but "distance" allowed me to deal with the issues myself. Even though I felt incredibly alone at times, I knew Henrietta really wasn't far away at all, and I was sure of her support and confidence.

I also encountered friends and resources I never knew were available. These experiences expanded my talents and interests, built my confidence, provided encouragement, and opened doors. My doctor was sensitive in helping unwed mothers prepare for labor and delivery. I even completed a semester of college classes while I was pregnant.

Through Henrietta's friends and acquaintances, I found out about programs that were available to single mothers. Another woman gave me part-time work I could do at home, so I could finish school and pay my medical expenses, and she opened doors for working and providing for my child.

Frankly, most of the days of my pregnancy were tough. But looking back I realize how good it was for me to be with Henrietta. She continuously loved, forgave, and enjoyed her family in spite of family ups and downs, and she set an example of endurance for me to love my family in the same way.

I've discovered that there are many seasons in life, and, depending on how you choose to deal with things, there can be something beautiful in every situation. As Henrietta would say, "Life's an adventure." By the grace and love of God, the support of my family, and the opportunity I had during pregnancy, I gradually came to a place of acceptance. As my baby grew, so did my love and strength. By the time my second beautiful, healthy girl was born, I was set in my decision to raise my child with goals and ideas in place.

To Parent or Not to Parent

Your friend is going to feel the impulses to choose parenting—they are the natural ones. (Ironically enough, the younger the mother, the more inclined she is to want to keep her baby.) But pray for wisdom for your friend, and help her to project as clearly as she can the future she can provide for the baby. Maybe, as in Lois's or Lorraine's cases, your friend is emotionally and financially prepared to begin a family. But many times, girls are not prepared to become single mothers.

I know of a social worker who stood on the steps of the hospital and cried as a penniless teenage mother who had decided to parent—despite her family's complete denial of any kind of shelter or support—rode away to a shelter for homeless women in the back of a police car. The baby was wearing clothes and a diaper the social worker had given the mother. Her tears were for the young mother as well as for her baby.

Ways to Help

1. Don't panic when your friend keeps changing her mind about parenting and adoption. Help her think ahead to explore all the possibilities.

2. If you have a long-range commitment to your friend, let her know you'll support her decision in practical ways. Be aware of your own feelings about whether your friend should parent. Remember that her decision is hers to make and will impact the rest of her life. Be more ready to listen than to advise.

3. Your friend may get excited about checking out all the details of a parenting budget, or she may not. The emotional and physical changes and tensions she's experiencing may make it hard for her to concentrate on details. Without being pushy, do everything you can to help her think ahead.

4. Again, encourage your friend to seek counsel.

7

All About Adoption

Adoption is your friend's alternative to choosing to parent her baby herself. To help her think clearly, you should familiarize yourself with what an adoption is all about.

Checking Out Adoptive Homes

Although many lawyers and doctors arrange independent adoptions with positive, healthy families, an agency is in an excellent position to select an adoptive home where the child will blend with the parents racially and physically, and to choose a family with a strong, positive home life. They screen couples regarding the strength of their marriage, their commitment to the future, and their commitment to each other. After examining education, reasons for wanting to adopt, financial situation, etc., agencies usually make at least one "home visit" to make sure a child placed in that home would be provided for adequately in every respect. When a girl considers an adoption plan for her coming baby, she can be assured that he will be placed in a secure, stable, two-parent home with a consistent, main caretaker (usually the wife) and with all the strengths, protection, and security that a husband/father can provide.

And here's the most wonderful part—a girl can be sure that her baby's adoptive parents will love and want that child. Usually they have yearned, searched, waited, and prayed for the baby for years. They are prepared to do their best for him—to parent him lovingly, to guide, encourage, and help him develop his unique talents and gifts. And also they will be able to meet his needs financially.

Agencies are extremely selective with prospective adoptive parents. The rules and processes vary from agency to agency and from state to state, but all agencies are careful to keep the best interests of the baby in the forefront of their policies.

Age requirements

Most agencies have age requirements for adoptive parents and siblings. Mine stipulates that both husband and wife must be no more than thirty-eight years older than the child they wish to adopt. A family with two children under five years of age will not be considered for a third child. The youngest child in the home must be at least eighteen months old at the time of application.

Siblings

If the social workers in my agency have placed one child in a childless home, they like to place another there eventually. My agency also tries to keep siblings together; however, this often results in difficult placement situations. Over the last twenty years, my agency has been involved with five sets of twins and has always placed each pair of twins together. Awhile ago the agency faced quite a challenge in placing a set of triplet babies and their three-year-old brother in the same home. The four spent a year and a half in three different foster homes—two of the triplets were together. Finally the agency placed all four with a childless couple, who assimilated them gradually over a few weeks, beginning with the two who had always been together. Now they are a complete family—all four children are still preschool-aged. Can you imagine their college costs in about fifteen years!?

Nineteen-year-old Kristin gave birth to a daughter she reluctantly released for adoption. Two years later she was pregnant again. She worked with the same counselor and again considered parenting and adoption. If she chose to release the baby, she wanted that second baby to go into the same home where her first baby had been adopted. The couple had not considered adopting another child, but under the special circumstances they were delighted to adopt Kristin's second baby.

Moms- and Dads-to-Be

Agencies typically require medical exams for each person in the adoptive home. A couple must turn in a physician's evaluation of the factors involved in a couple's inability to have children, if they are childless.

The agency will usually also evaluate a couple's marriage stability, relationship to each other, and reasons for wanting to adopt.

A couple doesn't have to own their own property, but their home must meet the state's minimum standards for safety and sanitation. Often, the adoptive mother is expected to remain at home with the adopted child for a certain period of time. And this is especially important when the adopted child is an infant or preschooler.

Family Study

After a review of the general requirements, the couple fills out an application, and an agency begins its "family study" or "home study." A case worker is assigned to follow through with that couple and the adoption. Usually the process takes a few months and includes one or two home visits. These studies help the agency decision-makers evaluate the readiness of couples to assume the responsibilities of adoptive parenthood.

The goal of the family study is to gain understanding and knowledge of the adoptive family in almost every area. The social worker and adoptive parents will discuss their personal histories, including childhood experiences, school and vocational adjustments, and emotional make-up. Sometimes couples are asked to write individual biographies. They talk about dating and courtship, and marital and family relationships. Even their most personal feelings about childlessness and motives for adoption are explored. The agency representative will talk with them about their feelings about illegitimacy and related areas, and a social worker will inquire about their experience with children.

In many agencies, an adoptive couple can indicate what type of child they want, whether boy or girl or medically needy. A social worker will ask if they would accept a baby whose birth mother was involved with drugs or alcohol.

The couple must furnish references from friends, employers, pastors, etc. They are even fingerprinted so the agency can make sure neither has a criminal record.

After the "inquisition," the counselor writes her lengthy report, and an approval team discusses any doubts or questions and makes the decision about the placement of a child. Either a couple is approved for adopting or recommended for future counseling.

And then the wait for the baby begins.

The Great Wait

Agencies vary a great deal in how long the couple must wait for a baby. The agency I work with only accepts twenty-five couples at a time, so almost every couple has a child within nine months or so after approval. When most of that set of twenty-five families have their babies at home, the agency takes on another twenty-five. So there are times when the intake at my agency is closed. This process eliminates years of suspenseful, frustrating waiting for couples who have been approved.

Now and then a difficult case comes up. One young birth mother who worked with my agency could not bring herself to sign the release papers. She did sign to place the baby in temporary foster care. Then she disappeared, and no efforts to find her turned up any clue. After four months, the agency started court proceedings to obtain custody of the child. But just as the time approached for the termination of that mother's rights, she phoned to inquire about her child and the court extended her rights. Then it happened again—and again; the child was left in limbo for three years. The agency felt certain they would eventually win the case, and so they placed the baby in a pre-adoptive home at eighteen months. That family eventually did adopt the little one who was already like their own. But what a precarious and uneasy time it was for those adoptive parents!

After the Adoption

Most agencies have a follow-up policy on all adoptions. My agency follows the couple and baby for six months to be sure that all is going well and that natural bonding has taken place. After the six-month period, the couple goes to court to finalize the adoption, and a new birth certificate is issued.

Following that court date, most agencies are no longer involved with the couple unless the couple wishes to maintain the relationship. Each year my agency sponsors an adoptive couples' retreat with various counselors and other professionals to teach and advise in helpful sessions, and all adoptive parents are invited.

Your Friend and the Adoption

You'll learn more about the pro's and con's of adoption for your friend in the next chapter, but it's good to understand how she fits into the process part of the adoption.

Most agencies spend a great deal of time and demonstrate concern for the birth mother as she approaches delivery, release, and adoption. Normally, she has received clear counsel and pre-natal classes during the months of her pregnancy. The classes are usually at the hospital where her baby will be born so that they will be expecting her and she can avoid the hassles of last-minute registration. The classes provide detailed instruction about the birthing process and how to cope with and participate in labor.

Her counselor (and in some cases, a foster-mother like me) will help prepare her for the hospital stay, explaining the onslaught of emotions that usually surround the experience. A birth mother may feel elated one day and depressed the next. A counselor will describe the post-partum depression that many women experience after delivering a baby so that the young mother will be prepared. Many of these mood swings are related to inevitable hormonal fluctuations, and a birth mother should try not to base long-range decisions about her baby's future on those feelings.

A birth mother's agency worker will also discuss the options she will have in the hospital. A girl can choose to see her baby a great deal, feeding and changing the child and taking pictures. Sometimes a birth mother facing the difficulties of releasing for adoption prefers to be moved out of the maternity section of the hospital and to see her baby less often or not at all. The counselor will talk with her about who will visit the birth mother in the hospital—parents, friends, the birth father? Does she have objections to having any of these people see the baby? Generally, counselors discourage friends from coming. The feelings and opinions they express can be conflicting and upsetting and often serve to confuse the young mother. Since the hospital stay is short, and she will be very tired anyway, lots of visitors are not a good idea.

Agencies vary in their policies for choosing adoptive families for a particular baby. In many agencies the birth mother chooses from a selection of current family profiles. The agency I work with allows a birth mother to study three family profiles before the baby's arrival, if she chooses. From the information of age, level of education, type of work, and type of personality, a young woman can choose the couple that will become her baby's parents.

Maureen chose a family from the profiles given to her. The ages of the adoptive parents were listed but not the birthdates. When the social worker called that family with the good news, she discovered that the baby had been born on the adoptive mother's birthday. The adoptive mother was delighted with that coincidence. And Maureen shed some happy tears over it, considering the surprise a confirmation of her choice. It helped ease the pain of parting.

While she was pregnant, Linda bought an outfit for her coming baby. She carefully embroidered a sailboat on the pocket, hat, and socks because she was a sailing enthusiast. Although it wasn't listed on the adoptive couple's profile, Linda's counselor discovered that the couple Linda had chosen loved to sail, too. Linda felt sure her baby was going to the right home!

Letters of Love

Many agencies permit birth mothers, if they choose, to send a gift with their babies. They are encouraged to write a letter to the child and to the adoptive parents; the letter to the child goes into a file at the agency (or, depending on the agency, into a file given to the adoptive parents), and the gift and letter to the parents go with the baby.

Darling, blue-eyed Kimberly became pregnant as a college student. Her parents were loving and supportive during this traumatic time. Kimberly was a talented girl; she played the piano well, wrote poetry, and liked to draw. During her time in the hospital with her newborn son, she made several sketches of him to send with the baby to his adoptive parents.

The following is Kimberly's letter to her son:

To my son,
You don't know me, but I love you.

I loved you from the moment I knew you existed in me, and that love will never die.

I love you so much. It broke my heart to give you up, but I felt it was best for both of us. I was single, and I didn't have a job—I wanted to give you everything I could, but it wouldn't have been enough. You deserved and needed a family—people who not only would love you with all their hearts, but who could also provide you with everything you would need.

It hurts. I look at the pictures of you and me in the hospital, and I know I will never stop loving you. You're a part of me . . . a very special part of me.

I pray you'll understand why I gave you up. I felt it was the *best* thing I could do.

Those few days in the hospital I held you close as often as I could. I fed you, I played with your tiny toes and fingers, I kissed you, I talked to you. You'd fall asleep holding onto my little finger. You were so precious. I wanted to keep you badly, but I knew in my heart it would be the wrong choice.

I pray for you every day. I pray that someday God will become a friend to you the way he has to me. I'm only making it through this by depending on his love and strength.

And I pray that your family is the best one you could ever have. I'm sure they are. I know they must love you very much.

They're the lucky ones—to see your first step, your first word, your first day of school. How I wish I could be there, how I wish I could be the one you call "Mom."

I know what I did was right for both of us, and I hope you'll be able to see it that way, too. I can understand how you may feel; I was also adopted. I know it can be puzzling. You may have questions and maybe feel a little pain, but I also know you don't have to feel angry or confused. For me it's just a fact, and, although I wonder sometimes, it doesn't hurt that my mother gave me up. My wonderful family loves me deeply, and that's what matters—being loved. Giving you up was the hardest, most painful thing I ever did. I love you.

Now I'm helping other single mothers who don't know what to do. You've been the inspiration of my recent poetry and artwork. You are in my thoughts constantly. Someday, when you have a child, you will understand truly what it is to look at your own flesh and blood. Imagine then how painful it would be to give your child away, although it is the best thing you can do, the only thing you can do. So much love along with so much sadness!

Good-bye now. Perhaps someday we'll meet—if not in this life, then in heaven with our Savior. Until then, my son, *always* know . . .

> I love you.

And here's Kimberly's letter to her baby's adoptive parents:

To my son's new parents:
He is my gift to you.

I know you will love him with all of your hearts, that you will take care of him the best you can. Raise him to know Christ, to be like Christ, to find his strength in him.

I pray for you, that you will stand in the hard and painful

times. You have my son now—he is yours. It hurts, but I know I've done the right thing. Through the experience I've grown closer to God and to my family.

They were behind me—my family. We are Christians, but—like all families—we have our sadnesses. We all love the baby. It has been difficult for them, too. I am adopted, too. My "birth" parents were college students—like me. My baby's father was not a college student. He had already graduated. He was handsome, but not very kind to me. He supported my decision to give our son up for adoption. I know he loved the baby in his own way.

It was hard. If my family hadn't been there I don't know what I would have done. I never could have aborted my son, but giving him up was harder than I knew, and I needed my family.

I love him very much. I write and draw about my son in my journal. I will always cherish him and love him. Having him is not something I will hide. Already there have been a few girls who have been encouraged by what I've done. Already God has made this something useful for his work.

It's strange. I didn't want to get pregnant, but now that I have been, I wouldn't change any of it. I loved him from the moment I knew he was inside me.

I know you love him, too—and I'm glad that I could give him to you. As I've said, he's *your* son now. Take care of yourselves and of him.

In Christ,
ME

The adoptive parents answered Kimberly's letter:

Dear Birth Mom,
Your letters to us were beautiful, and we'll always cherish them. The yellow gown and little dog are also special items we will

save for him. The prints you drew are absolutely wonderful. You have a special gift. We've shown them to everyone, and all have said how beautiful and special they are. We thank you for them. They'll hang in our home always. They are priceless to us.

We don't know how to thank you for another priceless gift. His name is Joshua David. We cherish him and love him, and we thank God for him. He is to us a miracle, a blessing bestowed only by the hand of God. We do realize the responsibilities of raising him. We will raise Joshua in our Christian faith, and he will grow to learn about and love his Lord. We dedicated him to the Lord this month. His name means "prosperous spirit."

I want to tell you a little about how he is doing. Joshua is a beautiful boy. He still has his dreamy blue eyes and dark hair. He smiles and laughs often. He loves music! His favorite time of day is when Daddy plays his guitar and we sing to him. He gets so excited! He also loves to watch me comb his hair in the mirror. He thinks he's just the most handsome guy around (and he gets no argument from us). Something else that we can't believe is that Joshua looks so much like his daddy. Everyone who sees Joshua says it's amazing how much they look alike. Daddy just *beams.*

Joshua is loved by everyone! Our families adore him, and grandparents are always making excuses to drop by or to babysit. Both sets live in town. Even his great-grandmother, eighty-seven years old, traveled a great distance to meet and hold him. One thing Joshua doesn't lack is love! He has a big sister named Laura. She is also adopted; we've had her since birth. She will be three in June. She is a terrific big sister. She calls Joshua "my baby" and is very protective of him. I'm sure they will have special things to share as they grow up together.

We remember you in our daily prayers and pray that you are

filled with the Spirit, encouragement, and joy. We can only imagine what is in your heart and all you have felt through this experience. You are a loving and very special person. I know God has a unique ministry at work in your life. We love you and continue our prayers for you and your family.

We love Joshua with every ounce of life and breath. He is a very happy and contented child, full of fun and loved by so many.

We hope and pray for peace in your life and nothing but the best.

God Bless You,
US

Many agencies have policies which allow a girl to receive one more letter from the adoptive parents and a picture of the baby during that first six months. Most adoptive parents are open and cooperative with my agency in this communication. The interchange helps the birth mother in the grieving process; she becomes reassured and more comfortable in her decision to release the baby, more confident that the agency has done its best to place her child in a loving home. It is a blessing to have enough information to picture the adoptive family, their home, their lifestyle. Although it doesn't erase the pain, it certainly makes it more bearable.

These first letters can be important. When one young mother was killed in a car accident a month after signing release papers, the agency contacted the baby's family so the adoptive parents could provide satisfying information someday for their child.

Depending on the state procedures, an adopted child eighteen or older who is interested in locating his birth mother can contact an agency. The agency continues to act as a go-between for the child and his birth mother. And when appropriate, when all the parties—adopted child, adoptive parents, and birth mother—agree, information may be released. For this reason, it is important for a birth mother to keep the agency informed of address changes.

When Sarah, an adopted child, turned eighteen, she returned to the agency I work with to find her birth mother. With the adoptive mom's full cooperation and support, the agency contacted the birth mom, who was willing and eager, and they all met. Now all three are friends—Sarah, her birth mother, and her adoptive mother. It's a very unusual, but lovely situation.

Other Priceless Gifts

Tammy sent a necklace of half a heart with her baby daughter. She kept the other half. Susan gave her baby a necklace that her own mother had worn as an infant. Susan had worn it, too. When her baby daughter grows up, that necklace will be a sure confirmation that her birth mother loved her and considered her most special.

Shelly made a scrap book for her baby, including the letter to her baby expressing her feelings and love. She put in pictures of the baby's father, Shelly's mom and dad, and pictures of Shelly with the baby in the hospital. No names were included, and the adoptive parents felt comfortable in keeping it for the little boy who might someday be happy to know what his birth parents and grandparents looked like.

Jean had a pair of her own baby shoes processed in ceramic with her baby's birthdate inscribed. She sent them along when she released her baby. Jean sends her daughter a birthday card every year. These cards are kept in a file at the agency I work with. If her daughter ever contacts the agency for information about her birth mother, she will be satisfied to know that her biological mother cared for and loved her through the years. Jean keeps an unusual diary about herself with pictures and events; she hopes it will bridge the gap of intervening years if her daughter ever comes seeking her.

A Lot to Think About

Your friend has a lot of information to assimilate right now. There are many ways you can help your friend, of course, but a good agency is the best resource for a pregnant young woman facing this tough circumstance. For her sake and the baby's sake, get all the information you can. The next chapter talks about some of the benefits and hurts associated with releasing a child for adoption.

* * *

Ways to Help

1. Be prepared with information about local adoption agencies and their policies regarding adoptive families and birth mothers.

2. If your friend is already planning to release her child for adoption, encourage her to work with a skilled counselor or social worker.

3. If she is planning to release her baby, make a long-range commitment to participate in her grieving process.

4. For more information about adoption, read some of the books listed in the resource section of this book.

5. Start praying for the right couple for your friend's child.

Legacy of an Adopted Child

Once there were two women
    Who never knew each other—
One you do not remember;
    The other you call Mother.

Two different lives
    shaped to make yours one—
One became your guiding star;
    The other became your sun.

The first gave you life,
    And the second taught you to live in it.
The first gave you a need for love,
    And the second was there to give it.

One gave you a nationality;
    The other gave you a name.
One gave you the seed of talent;
    The other gave you an aim.

One gave you emotions;
    The other calmed your fears.
One saw your first sweet smile;
    The other dried your tears.

One gave you up—
    It was all she could do.

The other prayed for a child,
   And God led her straight to you.

And now you ask me through your tears,
The age-old question through the years:
   Heredity or environment—
   which are you the product of?

Neither, my darling—neither.
   Just two different kinds of love.
                  Anonymous

8

Choosing Adoption

Whether an adoption is private (through a doctor and an attorney) or through an agency, the primary concern should center on the future of the child and his well-being. But there are issues regarding the birth mother that are important to keep in mind as well.

At first the idea of releasing her child for adoption may seem selfish and unnatural to you or to your friend. But depending on the situation, it might be the most unselfish, loving route your friend could take.

This difficult decision must be made carefully, because its consequences are lifelong for your friend and for her child. A counselor trained in helping young women decide between parenting and adoption is invaluable at this point. A counselor can help your friend consider how adoption benefits her future and also how releasing a child can hurt.

The Good Stuff

Depending on your friend's present living situation, releasing her baby could make a world of difference in her plans for the future.

Your friend may not be mature or prepared enough to take on the responsibility of childrearing. Waiting to parent may give her the time she needs to be the best parent she could be. Without a child, she would be free and more financially able to travel, develop relationships, and have some new experiences. These opportunities are even more important if your friend is young.

If your friend has not finished school, she would have the time and freedom to pursue education. Freedom to pursue a career or take a full-time job would provide a steady income for her and a satisfying work experience.

If your friend chooses to release her child for adoption, she will be free from the pain single mothers often experience when people make hurtful remarks about their situation. Your friend also would not face the difficulty of dating as a single mom or the fears surrounding the issue of how her baby would affect a future marriage. If she is very young and the family has been in turmoil over her pregnancy, sometimes the best way to preserve healthy family relationships is to release the child for adoption.

One of the positive feelings associated with an adoption release is the sense that the birth mother put her child's needs and future opportunities ahead of her own in an unselfish decision.

The Hard Part

When your friend chooses to release a baby for adoption, she is choosing loss and hurt. No baby is a "throw-away." That young mom bonds closely with her infant in those three days before she signs to release for adoption. The decision is a noble, costly sacrifice, and the young mother feels the hurt and separation deeply.

The grief is great. It will help prepare your friend to know beforehand what it might be like. Once again, this is where counsel becomes invaluable. Knowing beforehand and understanding the feelings that will assault her after she signs the release papers will help equip your friend to cope, to move through her feelings, and eventually to accept the loss.

Some knowledge of the grief process may be helpful to you in interpreting your friend's reactions and in helping her get through the difficult time. Remember that stages are fluid. Your friend may move back and forth between the stages—that's normal. She may feel some, all, or more than the feelings we will cover in these pages. Above everything else, treat your friend with patience and gentleness during this time and help her to be patient and gentle with herself!

The following are some of the reactions associated with the grieving process that your friend may go through.

Denial/Shock

For awhile, your friend may "stick her head in the sand," so to speak. This reaction becomes a defense against painful reality. She may do and say things you've never seen her do and say before. The general attitude is something like, "The whole thing never really happened." This stage cannot last long; reality is insistent! Eventually your friend will express other emotions.

Sadness/Depression

Your friend may go through days when she feels she carries a giant lump in her throat—a lump that feels as big as a grapefruit. The grief of the experience is always right there at the surface. She may exhibit the general symptoms of depression: low energy and apathy, sleeping too much, eating too little or too much, and other physical symptoms. She may burst into tears while watching television (Pampers commercials, and other programming and advertising that put babies on screen) or when encountering a pregnant person.

She may feel guilt. It's easy to forget the wisdom of the decision in the moments when she thinks of her very own child in someone else's home. And very likely she will experience loneliness, because no one (except the Lord!) can know exactly the depth of her grief and emotion.

Anger

Your friend may feel angry inside—at herself, at family members who hurt more than helped, at the father of her baby, at the adoption agency or the adoptive parents, at God, and at the world that seemed to allow such painful experiences. Her anger may even show up in a grumbling, simmering irritability, or in moments of very strong, rage-like anger.

Such a reaction is normal. Be patient during these times. Don't take her anger too personally. You may be a big help in keeping her from making any major decisions during those times of intense anger.

Fear/Bargaining with God

Your friend will always, always live with second thoughts. "Did I really do the right thing?" "If only . . ." Believe it or not, the young woman who chooses to parent her child asks these same questions. She may doubt or mistrust her decision. "Are my baby's adoptive parents really as wonderful as they sound?" She may pass many moments in wishful thinking, "If only I had been financially stable . . ." "If only I had been a bit older . . ." If only the baby's father . . ."

This can be a dangerous time for your friend's faith, if she is a Christian, because it's easy to misunderstand God's character of love, especially if she has never experienced that love for herself. She may be tempted to pray "let's make a deal" prayers like: "God, if you'll do this for me, I'll . . ." You can be an enormous help during this time. Pray for wisdom, asking God to help you understand your friend's fears and spiritual struggles.

Persistence

Although she has experienced great trauma, your friend may actually go through a period when she is unwilling to let go of the sadness and the feelings of loss. She may feel she is cutting herself off from her baby if she releases her grief or comes to a place of acceptance. A whole new feeling of guilt for abandoning the pain arrives. Help your friend to see that the negative feelings are not her only connection to her child. Help her both to struggle and to hope.

Acceptance

This stage of your friend's process will be a joyful time for you, too, as you watch her relax in a new peace and comfort after being so close to her pain. At this stage your friend becomes comfortable (not necessarily *happy*) with the decision she made and will feel peace about her experience. Those days of the "grapefruit" lump in her throat will be behind her now.

As you watch your friend travel in and out of these stages, commit yourself to pray for her daily and to spend time with her. The varying factors of family emotional support sometimes make the grieving process even more difficult for certain young women. Be an unwavering support during this rocky period.

I Can Do All Things

Here's what one young birth mother had to say about the circumstances surrounding the release and adoption of her baby.

When I discovered I was pregnant, my parents helped me seek a solution to the dilemma. I wasn't married, and the father of my child was not interested in me anymore. I wanted to give my baby up for adoption from the very beginning since I felt that having two mature parents was important.

We came across an agency that helped girls like me. I was assigned a counselor. Everyone was friendly and supportive. I came to live with Henrietta, who became a real friend for the next four months. She was kind and helpful, but best of all, she listened. I felt she had complete trust and confidence in me. Though this was an extremely difficult time, her influence helped me to use my faith in the Lord, and he *did* help me. I had regular sessions with my counselor, and she helped me to reach a healthy attitude and to cope with my problem.

I also got a job with a real estate appraiser who was a Christian. He and his wife were patient and kind, and the job itself was good therapy—the long hours of waiting were filled with productive work.

I thank God for that job and those wonderful people he sent to help me with this struggle. I also thank him for delivering me from the agony and suffering that many go through when giving up a child for adoption. When I recall that hard time, a scripture comes to mind: "I can do all things through Christ, who strengthens me."

"Get That Baby Back!"

Remember Sandy from the beginning of this book? She was the first girl who stayed with me during a pregnancy. One day a friend of hers called me. Melissa was a college student and four months pregnant. "Henrietta, I want to stay with you and have Sandy's doctor and place my baby in a family—just like Sandy did." But her mother didn't agree; she wanted Melissa to have an abortion, and the pressure at home was becoming intolerable.

I sent Melissa information about my agency. I felt it was best for her to work through the agency, which provided counseling and pre-natal training. It didn't take her long to make a decision.

"I'm coming, okay?" I had other pregnant girls living with me at the time, but of course it was okay. She came in her own car, traveling a thousand miles alone. How that pretty, blonde bundle of energy sparked up my household! She enrolled in two courses at our local junior college: creative writing and—heaven help us—racquetball!

"Racquetball? Melissa!" I was worried about the baby, but had to laugh. "Check with Dr. Jim, okay?"

Dr. Jim told her to go ahead, but not to overdo it. As the classes continued, the class members had competition matches between them. Melissa beat everyone in the class—and most of them were guys. She had a terrific time, but how humiliating it must have been for all those guys to be beaten by a girl, five and a half months pregnant!

Her writing was imaginative and creative—her teacher encouraged her to seek publication. She kept a daily journal about her health and thoughts and feelings. Since she was positive her baby would be a girl, she named her and talked to her on the pages of her notebook. She often shared snatches from her journal with me, and I enjoyed her open-heartedness. (When her baby *boy* was born, she said, "I'm keeping the name. It's not that girlish—I can't change the whole journal!")

She borrowed my boxed set of the *Chronicles of Narnia.* "Wow—I've read these one at a time over the years, but wouldn't it be great to read them straight through? If it's okay, I'm going to stay in my room and read all day—I'll come out for supper!" she exclaimed. And she did. She read for three days, only coming out to eat with us. I almost envied that total immersion in C.S. Lewis's fantasies. But I don't think I'll ever come up with three full days to do it!

The situation with Melissa's mother remained difficult. When Melissa left home her mother said, "Don't tell me when that baby is born. Don't tell me what sex it is. Don't tell me anything about the birth. Just come home when it's all over." She wasn't so much angry as hurting herself. Her inability to cope with the hurt and the loss made her seem completely disinterested. She encouraged Melinda to come home to finish her education at a local college but under no circumstances to consider bringing the baby home.

Even without her mother's ultimatum, Melissa never considered keeping her child. She even confessed to me, "I'm not very fond of kids!" When her newborn son was placed next to her on the delivery table, she looked at him for a few moments then looked up at me. "Am I less of a woman because I don't love him?" she asked.

I hugged her. "You're not less of anything—except pregnant! Let's talk about it tomorrow." She had prepared her mind to release that baby, and in those first few moments she was not going to attach herself to that little son who wouldn't always be hers.

But when I arrived the next day, coming through the door with flowers and a book, she chattered on and on of nothing but that baby boy! "He's so precious, so helpless, so perfect!" Melissa was head-over-heels in love with him.

Since Melissa wanted to be involved in the choice of her son's adoptive home, the agency gave her the profiles of three couples who had been approved and were waiting for a child. She chose a family who enjoyed camping, canoeing, and backpacking—she wanted her little boy to grow up enjoying the great outdoors as much as she did.

It was Good Friday afternoon when I picked up Melissa from the hospital. She sobbed and sobbed on the way home. The pain of separation was acute. Finally I stopped the car and held her close.

"Oh, Melissa," I said tenderly, "you've sent your firstborn away from your bosom. Seeing you suffer is giving me a great big, new appreciation for what it cost our heavenly Father to send his Son all the way to earth. Your loss is the gift of a good life to your baby, but God sent his Son knowing that Good Friday was ahead for him. I'll never forget you, Melissa, or what you're teaching me today!"

The next few days were sad. She signed the release papers the next morning (after the required seventy-two hours were up). On Sunday, which was Easter, Melissa's mom called and talked on and on about trivial things. After about twenty minutes I slipped Melissa a note: "Aren't you going to tell her about the baby?" Melissa shook her head. At the end of her long, one-sided conversation, her mom said, "Well, Melissa, let me know when it's all over and you're fine."

"It's already all over, Mom, and we're both fine," Melissa replied.

At this point her mother fell apart, crying and saying, "Did you sign the papers? Why didn't you call me!? I didn't mean all those

things I said to you. *Get that baby back!* You can bring him home."
She was nearly hysterical when she hung up the phone.

Her mother's hysterics and unpredictable change of attitude
regarding the baby didn't help Melissa much. Some counseling
with her mother earlier in Melissa's pregnancy would have helped.
Melissa had enough to cope with in her own sadness! She confided
to me that twice she had put her hand on the phone to call her
mother and beg for permission to bring her baby boy home. But
she had to remove that hand with the other hand forcibly to keep
herself from making the call. She cried, and we talked about it.

"Perhaps God didn't want that phone call to happen. I know
your mom has had a hard time with your pregnancy, but I'm
feeling pretty angry with her just now," I said honestly. "She's had
six months to deal with the arrival of this baby, and she has denied
her interest in your pregnancy and the baby all along. But she
really *did* care. Now she's heaping her own grief on you, forgetting
that you have pain of your own to bear. What if you brought him
home, and she changed her mind in three months?"

"Oh, you're right!" Melissa sobbed. "She's awfully changeable.
It couldn't have worked out."

"Call your counselor, Melissa. She won't mind that it's Easter.
Talk with her about it."

Melissa's counselor spent half an hour on the phone with her.
She encouraged Melissa to take some time alone in her room to go
over all the reasons she had written down both for keeping her
baby and for releasing him. "I'll come in the morning, and we'll
talk," she promised.

Before that morning appointment, Melissa's mother called
again. "I'm seeing a lawyer today. You see one up there, and *get
that baby back!*" Melissa's mother was frantic over the loss of her
grandchild—an understandable response. But her ultimatums
were making Melissa's struggle over releasing the baby even
harder to bear.

"I'll let you know, Mom," Melissa said.

After a long morning session with her counselor, Melissa considered her dilemma all day without talking about it much. In the evening she called her mom. "Mom, my decision is a good one. I'm doing it for him because I love him so much. I'll be home in two weeks." Then she hung up.

In the months that Melissa lived with us, my son Jeff and Melissa had become good friends. He'd visited her in the hospital and even given her a live baby bunny when she came home. She was amused and somehow comforted by Jeff's thoughtfulness. A tiny rabbit to love is not a complete comfort for the pain of separating from her child, but that bunny provided an outlet for her tender feelings and affections. She carried that bunny all over the house (in a towel to avoid any mishaps!), holding it and playing with it. And that bunny traveled the thousand miles home with her.

She called me the next Easter weekend (that first birthday of a released child is so difficult). Now she's finishing her college courses and working part-time. And she's coping beautifully.

Not Only Melissa

The release of a baby was not just hard for Melissa. It's hard for every birth mother. I know a young social worker who says she is grateful for the bathroom adjoining her office. "It's important for days when a birth mother signs her release papers. I stay cool and together while I'm with my client so I can support her, but afterward I hide in there and share her tears."

But *hard* doesn't mean *bad* or *impossible*. The extent of the sacrifice and loss just makes the gift of a loving, two-parent home an even greater gift of love.

Stick by your friend in the weeks, months, even years after the release of her baby. That grieving period is her neediest time!

* * *

Ways to Help

1. Encourage your friend to make a list of the benefits to herself if she releases her baby for adoption.

2. Encourage your friend to list the benefits to her child if she releases her baby for adoption.

3. When you can, talk with your friend about the various stages of grieving to help her recognize and deal with them. Be prepared to cry with her. Don't minimize her grief by reminding her how happy the adoptive parents are.

4. Allow her to talk about her baby, remember her baby's name, and remember the baby's birthday with her. Keep on loving her!

9

Great Expectations—and Real Life!

There's no doubt about it—involvement in ministering to other people is one of the most exciting parts of life. But ministry can be hard work, too. And it's the disappointments and struggles that challenge us to love more and to commit more deeply. This time of unexpected pregnancy may be the hardest of your friend's life, so no doubt it will also hold some frustration and tears for you, her friend. Don't give up when the going gets tough; the rewards for sticking to it are infinite!

I've loved working with the young women who have stayed with me during these last few years—beginning with Sandy, who won my heart to this particular type of service. And I've grown and changed and stretched my ability to be flexible and to communicate love to a wide variety of girls.

Some of the girls who have lived with us have been a delight; others were difficult. But all of them were worth the time and effort expended. Through my experiences with these very different girls, I've learned a great deal about how families, friends, and their home environments shaped their behavior, and I have learned to trim down my expectations of their conduct.

Houserules

Before they come to live with me, the young ladies read, agree to, and sign a set of guidelines. Really, these few rules are quite lenient, but they give me a basis for discussion if they are violated excessively.

One of the established guidelines is that they clean their rooms and bathroom once a week and that they cook one meal a week for the whole "family." Jennifer was one of my difficult girls. She loved to cook but never cleaned anything! I tried some gentle pressure. I bought more clothes hangers and handed her a dozen, saying, "I know your closet is short of hangers, Jennifer. Here are some extras so you will have a place for some of the things on the floor." My own teenagers would have required nothing more than that hint. But not Jennifer! The next week, when we were in a light mood and she was playing pool with Jeff, I said, "Jennifer, you haven't cleaned your room yet. Why do you wait? Do you *like* living in that mess?"

Jennifer snapped back at me, "What about Jeff's room?" Fortunately, her remark struck me as funny—I have a pretty good sense of humor.

"Agreed!" I laughed. "His room isn't the best either. But you signed an agreement when you came here to live that you would keep your room clean. Jeff didn't sign anything when he arrived!"

We all laughed together, but even that didn't push her to clean her room.

Jennifer's birthday was the following week. I had turned the other girl living with me into a spy to discover Jennifer's favorite cologne and had bought her some. Since the girls are away from their families, we make a big deal out of their birthdays with dinners, banners, balloons, and gifts. That Sunday we were all in the kitchen cooking Sunday dinner together when I discovered I needed something stored in a drawer in Jennifer's room.

I was appalled when I stepped into the room—there were dust balls under the bed and all over the floor. Spider webs with tiny spiders in them lurked in the corners. Clothes were strewn everywhere, and the whole room smelled foul!

I returned to the kitchen and said quietly, "Jennifer, this is just not fair. My home is beautiful, and I have done my best to make you feel comfortable and welcome here. But now one corner of my home looks like a pig sty."

Her reply couldn't have shocked me more if she had slapped me: "Listen, that is MY room—when the door is closed, YOU STAY OUT!"

Lessons Learned

I went to my room to cry alone. The day was completely ruined; there was no dinner, no party, no present for Jennifer. I spent the next few hours weeping in frustration, anger, and hurt. How could she be so ungrateful? Her folks were not even paying for her food, let alone anything else. Everything was being provided for her, even her maternity clothes.

I called her counselor the next day to talk about resigning from the agency. I felt inadequate and resentful and ineffective. That wise counselor insisted that we have a conference in her office— me, Jennifer, and the other girl living with us.

"Okay, we're all going to say what's truly on our hearts, starting with you, Henrietta," she said.

I told her about the day before, what had been said, how I reacted, how the birthday was ruined. "I still have Jennifer's wrapped gift in my room. But I don't even feel like giving it to her," I said.

"I really thought the Lord wanted me to do this work. I was so enthusiastic about it! But I think I read the road signs the wrong way. I don't think I'm qualified or capable enough. I don't know how to handle this kind of difficulty, and I don't think I want to," I confessed.

The counselor had to pass a box of tissues around. The girls were crying, and so was I. Jennifer was next, and I was so surprised by her comments.

"I know I was awful, but it was my birthday. I didn't even want to be in her house. I just wanted to be home with my family," she admitted.

But Jennifer! I thought, *your family is a mess!* She was the fourth of six children. Her father had left the family but lived nearby with another woman. Her mom worked and had a live-in boyfriend. Her sixteen-year-old brother beat Jennifer up, and her junior-high aged sister had her own key to the house and kept very late hours. I was learning an important lesson: Although they were a fractured family, they were *hers* and she loved and missed them.

I had expected gratitude from the girls who lived in my lovely, comfortable home. But gratitude is a learned attitude, an attitude that needs to be taught and practiced, and many homes don't provide that instruction. I trimmed my expectations. I no longer miss something I don't expect.

Bless that counselor! The girls and I went home friends, ready to try again. And we celebrated a belated birthday! Jennifer started back to school while she lived with me—a tough place to be after having dropped out two years earlier. She was older than the other kids, the school was unfamiliar and she had no friends, and her pregnancy was becoming very obvious. It was tough, but she stuck it out and received her diploma. Jennifer kept her baby, even though she could not return to her family and would have to receive Public Aid. I have not heard from her again.

It's easy to form great expectations of how your area of ministry will develop, but it's even more wonderful to be part of the sometimes difficult process of how God works in human lives—yours and others'.

Do you feel that you are "expecting" something from your pregnant friend? Do you "expect" her to choose for her baby what you think you would choose if you were in her position? Do you "expect" heartfelt gratitude? Then trim down your expectations. You won't miss what you don't expect, and you'll be delighted when your friend *does* respond with warmth and enthusiasm to your interaction in her life.

Culture Shock

Twenty-year-old Pat came to me from a large city where she lived in a changing, but not violent, neighborhood. She told me many things about her life that made my heart ache for her. Pat was number seven out of eight children. Before she was born, when her parents had only five children, Pat's father fell ill and had to be hospitalized for six months. Pat's mom couldn't provide for or look after the children, so she released the older four to the state for adoption, keeping only the baby boy. After Pat's father came home, they had three more daughters. When her older brother was seven, the state removed him from their home because of child abuse. Eventually he too was released for adoption.

When Pat was eight, her father left the family. No one felt it a great loss because of his alcoholism. With the help of Public Aid, Pat's mom and the three girls eked out an existence. At fourteen, Pat and her mother argued bitterly over the boys Pat dated until eventually her mother told her to leave the house and never come back. Pat became an official ward of the state and lived in a group home until she turned eighteen.

Pat drifted between low-paying jobs and cut-rate hotels. All her possessions were contained in two battered suitcases. Since the weekly rent at her "hotels" was due on Mondays, Pat had established a pattern of having to move by the fourth week of each month because the month's welfare money was used up by the third week. A girlfriend's couch or a shelter for the homeless would carry her through until the next Public Aid check arrived. She was one of many living such a precarious, nomadic existence.

When she discovered she was pregnant, someone put her in touch with my agency, and she came to me during the last three months of her pregnancy. She stole a friend's radio to pawn it for the train fare into the suburbs, then she carefully mailed the pawn ticket back to him so he could redeem his radio. For her, it was the honorable thing to do. For me, it was a glimpse into an unfamiliar culture.

Pat was a new experience for me. She cared little for the cleanliness of her surroundings, although she was personally clean. She didn't enjoy my acres of grass and trees, but missed the city with its bustling crowds and stores for window shopping. "Your yard is just too neat. I'd like to take a garbage bag full of tin cans and paper and strew them around," she said. I spent my days with Pam in "culture shock"—she surprised me with each day's new comments and attitudes.

She also smoked a pack of cigarettes a day, although we talked about the danger for her baby. I didn't want to make a big deal out of the smoking, because Pat had much bigger problems to cope with. However, I didn't allow her to smoke inside the house. So Pat sat on the front step to smoke and flipped her cigarette butts into my bed of petunias. After four days I discovered quite an accumulation of butts in the flowers outside my front door.

"Pat," I said, "I'll get you an empty coffee can for your butts—they really don't look very nice among the flowers. Could you be helpful and pick them up?"

"You're too fussy," she said without moving.

"All right. I'll pick them up this time," I said, praying for a large dose of Job's patience, "but don't throw any more there."

I had to ignore the smoking problem so I could make an attempt at some of the other obvious needs in Pat's life. She especially needed to talk and talk and talk about her past—her father, her mother, her sisters. "The reason I am the way I am is because my mother never loved me," she stated.

I agreed with her that her past had been unusually difficult. "But those things are behind you now. How can we concentrate on the future?" We discussed types of jobs or job training she might pursue.

"Aw, it's too late for all of that!" Pat said.

My heart was heavy. Imagine—what would it be like to be devoid of hope at age twenty?

Once she said to me, "I don't trust anyone."

"What about me? You can trust me, Pat," I replied.

Her answer was startling. "How do I know that?"

And I had to agree she really didn't.

The Hard Truth

Pat's time with me was particularly difficult because I felt unable to help her enough. Of course I couldn't turn back time to give her a different father, mother, and sisters. I couldn't undo a lifetime of hurt with a few months of love and encouragement. The hard truth was, I couldn't do *anything* to help Pat in the areas where she needed it most. It was easy to become discouraged.

You may feel discouraged right now, too. Your friend has at least one problem that you can't solve for her—the unplanned pregnancy. And maybe she has others like Pat's that you long to "undo" or fix with your love. Don't focus on what you *can't* accomplish for your friend. Find some encouragement in doing what you *can* do.

You can't make your friend choose life for her unborn child, but you can put together some materials for her to read or to read with her. You can't receive her family's hurt and anger for her, but you can provide family-type support and encouragement during this tense time. No matter how much you love her, you can't take away her memories of a child given up to an adoptive family, but you *can* remember along with her, participating in the sorrow and the hope and the prayers for her future and the future of her child.

I couldn't take away Pat's long history of hurt, but I could add a period of acceptance and support to that life history. At my house, Pat wasn't ignored, neglected, or kicked out. At my house, she was not abused or criticized. I couldn't change the problems of the past, but it was within my power to limit the problems of the present.

So focus on what you can do, and be glad for whatever form those helpful actions take. Sometimes it's the small things that communicate a big love!

Ways to Help

1. Do something special for your friend that has nothing to do with her pregnancy—something that affirms her as a person. Remember her birthday, or bake a cake and take it to her house for no reason at all. Surprise her with a flower or a card.

2. With your actions, remind her that you remember she's a regular person and not just an unwed, pregnant person. Visit her the way you did before she was pregnant. Go shopping together. See a movie. Talk with her about your own struggles and joys.

3. Do you have any "great expectations" of your friend? Are they reasonable or unreasonable? Can you adjust them or put them on hold during this crisis time?

10

A Better Way

One of the most important, lasting contributions you can make to your friend's well-being is to help her, throughout her crisis experience, to shape a new perspective and value system regarding love and sex.

Maybe you're thinking, "The last thing my friend needs is someone else to preach at her!" And you're absolutely right. But you *can* help her think through these issues without "preaching" or forcing your personal ethical code on her.

Words We've Almost Forgotten

Hardly anyone uses the word "chastity" anymore. Maybe you don't even know what the word means; the dictionary defines it as *purity*—or *virtue*, another lovely word. It means moral excellency or goodness. How ironic that words of such beauty and the actions of value they represent should become almost obsolete in today's society! We've replaced moral excellence and goodness with moral decay at all levels of our society: in Washington, DC, in our community leadership, in our universities and high schools, in our businesses—yes, and even in our churches, Boy Scout Troops, and daycare centers.

The value systems of our parents and grandparents are mocked. No one can delineate right or wrong anymore. We base our decisions on whims. "If it feels good, do it!" and "If it gets me where I want to go, why not lie, cheat, and steal? Who's going to tell me not to?" are the mottos of the day. When a young person confesses his virginity, he is belittled, disbelieved, or pressured to "get with it." No wonder they call it the "me" generation—self is the standard.

Today I see all the evidences of what Francis Schaeffer has called "a post-Christian era." We're living in it. And what about sexual "freedom"? We've got it, all right, and like everyone else teens have bought into it, developing an unusually promiscuous sexual lifestyle.

Dismantling the Great Lie

The freedom of "if it feels good, do it" initially appeals to any young person, but is "sexual freedom" really *free*? Ask your friend. Ask any of the thirty-two pregnant girls who have lived with me; they would describe an exorbitant physical and emotional price. Ask the agency that worked with my thirty-two girls and hundreds of others to add up the costs of counseling hours, office hours, emotional input, and hospital and doctor bills. Ask the parents and family members of a young woman in crisis pregnancy about the cost in finances and in emotional strain. Can anyone put a price on never knowing or being involved in the life of a first child or grandchild? Ask a girl with raging herpes who has to deliver her child by Caesarean section to protect the baby's health, incurring large surgical bills which she has no resources to pay.

Ask a girl who aborted her baby how "free"—from pain, guilt, cash, or far-reaching emotional and physical consequences—her experience has been.

"Sexual freedom" is a misnomer. It has its own price tag, and the price is steep. But we don't see these negatives when we turn on the TV, or open a grocery-store novel, or pay attention to the advertising that we encounter every time we turn around. The media tells a lie, or at the very least, a half-truth. The media's projected roads all seem to lead to the bedroom, and the way is lined with glamour and glitz and sweetness and tenderness. Why ruin such a pleasant fantasy by thinking about the next morning, the following week, or the lifetime ahead?

The lie is summed up in two completely false equations: Sex = Love and Love = Sex. We believe the lie ourselves, without even realizing it. We pass it on to those around us. But sexual freedom is *not* free, and we must learn to exchange the lie with this truth: Sex = sex and produces an *illusion* of love. Love, the real thing, is much more elusive.

"I love French fries" doesn't even come within range of, "I love my wife more today than the day we married!" A young man's urgent, pleading, "But I love you, so it's all right to go all the way," is a far cry from, "I love you, so I'll wait to give you the best."

The most sinister lies closely resemble the truth. A young man's tender words and physical yearning really do look like "the real thing," especially when a young woman is longing for that once-in-a-lifetime love. It takes a great deal of courage for her to probe and test his promises of love without gambling her chastity.

Everyone Is Doing It

"Everyone is doing it" is another clever deception. One of the greatest pressures in our culture, and especially in the teen context, is to conform, to be part of the "in-crowd." And this deception is almost true—a whole lot of people—most, in fact—*are* "doing it."

But not everyone! Statistics show that 65-80 percent of young people will have experienced sex by the time they reach twenty years of age. And Christian teens fall only ten percentage points behind the secular statistic (*Why Wait*, p. 99). But 75 percent is not everyone. The 25 percent who champion chastity still form a significant minority.

Help your friend think through some of the "prizes" that the 75 percent have gained through their pursuit of sexual liberty. Pregnancy isn't the only "prize" that can result from casual sex. Let's explore some of the long-range problems.

Rejection

Young people face rejection when the partners to whom they have become so emotionally attached and physically joined move on to someone else. Remember the statistic regarding breakups in a crisis pregnancy situation? Ninety-five percent of those relationships don't make it, even if the problem pregnancy was "solved" by abortion. In 98 percent of the cases in which a girl carries a baby to term, the father of her child is already involved with someone else before the baby is born. And from that slim percentage of those who do marry because of a crisis pregnancy, the failure rate of those marriages reaches 90 percent in the first six years (Brandsen, p. 7).

The lie promises enduring love and pleasure; the rejection is the great surprise. A girl who gave in to sexual pressure because she feared her boyfriend would leave her suffers a rejection far more deep and damaging to her person when he does leave her.

An illusion of love

Casual sex offers a shabby imitation of the real thing. Sex without commitment is a gross misappropriation of God's great gift. God created the whole system of sexual pleasure and procreation to operate within the framework of married love. True love involves the binding of two personalities in a lasting relationship on *every* level: spiritual, intellectual, emotional, and physical. And sexual intimacy is an ultimate expression of that binding together. To settle for anything else is to cheat ourselves and the other people involved.

Promiscuity

Sexual activity, once begun, is nearly impossible (not completely impossible—we'll talk about that later) to stop.

Low self-esteem

Casual sex belittles both partners. It sends a message, "You are worth something if—and only if—you sleep with me. You are not worth my exertion to discipline myself to wait for you." Think about the locker room boasts of casual sex: the more conquests, the more "macho." Does mentioning a girl's name in that context bring her honor? Does it express love? Certainly not. It expresses lust. Promiscuity leads to a loss of self-respect and respect for one's partner.

Almost every young person struggles with self-esteem. But these ultimate needs for approval, popularity, and a sense of "belonging" cannot be met through a sexual encounter with another person involved in the same struggle.

Your friend's self-esteem is determined by who she is—not by what she does or has done. She is valuable! God created her unique, a "one-of-a-kind" person. He loved her as he planned her and gave her potential beyond her wildest dreams.

Another person's immature assessment will change with the winds. But God's opinion won't. And he's the only one who counts.

Disease

Some of that 75 percent will find themselves entrapped in the quicksand of our society's escalating problem with sexually-transmitted diseases. The statistics regarding the spread of these diseases are not simply doubling and tripling; they are increasing exponentially.

At the forefront of current media representation is AIDS—the Acquired Immune Deficiency Syndrome. This problem had been mainly confined to sexually active homosexuals, but it has spread into the heterosexual population. One researcher expressed his horror at the advancement of the disease: "We have more heterosexuals infected today than we had homosexuals infected five years ago" (*Why Wait*, p. 206).

AIDS is quickly becoming the number one public health problem of the world. Dr. C. Everett Koop, Surgeon General of the United States, recently said, "After more than half a century in medicine, I can say that nothing is more frightening to me than the specter of AIDS in the future of public health." And 70 percent of the ever-increasing number of babies born with AIDS die within six months (*Why Wait*, p. 207).

The disease is frightening and mysterious; there is no cure, and treatment helps very little. Carriers may never experience any symptoms of the disease, so they may spread AIDS without realizing it. The period of incubation (the length of time before the disease evidences itself) is so long that victims sometimes can't even recall who the carrier was. And the disease is ugly. AIDS is extremely debilitating; it wastes its victims to skeletons.

The Secretary of Health and Human Services recently remarked, "If our predictions are correct for global statistics, fifty million up to one hundred million could die from AIDS by the end of the century." Obviously, the problem is not unique to the United States. AIDS is rampant in Central Africa; between 9 and 11 percent of the entire population is infected (*Why Wait*, p. 207).

Although there are no teenagers with AIDS (except those who received contaminated blood during a transfusion), the disease's incubation period is somewhere between five and fifteen years. An infection from their high-school years may not show up until they reach their twenties and thirties.

There are other ways AIDS is transmitted. A brilliant young intern accidentally cut through his glove and skin while operating on an AIDS patient. When he contracted the disease, he lost his career as well as his health. A lab technician acquired the virus through a scratch on her hand while working with the blood of an AIDS patient. Many dentists now wear protective surgical gloves. But the overwhelming majority of AIDS victims contracted the virus through sexual contact.

And AIDS is just one of many sexual-transmitted diseases. There are more than twenty-seven known to the medical profession. Some, if diagnosed, can be treated and corrected; others, such as genital herpes, have no cure. Mothers and unborn babies form a high-risk population. Low birth weight, premature birth, infertility, infections, retardation, and blindness are a few of the problems doctors fear when a young mother is infected with a sexually-transmitted disease.

Certainly it's true that condoms are better than nothing. But a condom is not a guarantee. Some women have contracted the AIDS virus while depending on a condom for protection.

Think About the Future

That remnant of sexually inactive single people have the right idea: chastity! Playing with casual sex is playing with fire.

Help your friend ask these tough questions: Am I risking my future marriage by being sexually active now? Am I risking my own future physical and emotional health by being sexually active now? Am I risking the health of my "someday" children? Am I risking infertility? What elements of "the lie" did I fall for? Which of the results of casual sex have I experienced?

I mentioned earlier that sexual activity is hard to let go of once it's begun. And it is hard, but not impossible. Remember Anne, the girl whose boyfriend Dave was so supportive during her pregnancy? A few months before her recent marriage to another young man, Marty, she talked about a "second virginity"—an ability to feel that all things were new and that she could withstand the temptation to become sexually involved outside of marriage. "I know without a doubt that God has forgiven me. It's been like starting over," she said. "I'm so glad I've had the chance to honor both Marty and the Lord by waiting until we're married for sex."

The results of past sexual behavior cannot be undone. But God's promise is true: "If anyone is in Christ, he is a new creation" (2 Corinthians 5:17). Encourage your friend with hopes for her future.

The Best Is Yet to Be

The best reason to steer clear of sexual activity outside of marriage is that God—who made you, your partner, and the universe and knows what's wise—calls it foolish and dishonoring to him.

Help your friend aim high—at the kind of enduring love that God describes in his Word:

> Love is patient, love is kind. It does not envy, it does not boast, it is not proud. It is not rude, it is not self-seeking, it is not easily angered, it keeps no record of wrongs. Love does not delight in evil but rejoices with the truth. It always protects, always trusts, always hopes, always perseveres. Love never fails.
> *1 Corinthians 13:4-8a*

* * *

Ways to Help

1. Encourage your friend to think about her definitions of love and her attitudes about sex. Does she believe Love = Sex and Sex = Love? Help her shape a new perspective and a new value system to guide future relationships.

2. Bring up the topic of "sexual freedom." Talk about the possible positives and negatives.

3. If your friend is struggling with low self-esteem, encourage her. Affirm her value to you and her value to God.

4. Pray for your friend, that she will be able to stand strong in future times of sexual temptation.

11

Where Do You Go From Here?

Maybe you'd never considered the widespread problem of crisis pregnancy until your friend became pregnant. Now that you've assimilated some facts and are working through this difficult time with your friend, you may be wondering how you can use this experience in further ministry opportunities. *Feeling* interested and convicted about a problem is a good thing; finding concrete ways to help is even better!

Be Informed

Maybe, in helping your friend, you've already begun to accumulate a stockpile of information. The helping pro-life ministries listed in the back of this book provide a jumping-off place for becoming informed.

Articles and books that explore crisis pregnancy, abortion, adoption, and single parenting are being written all the time. Stay alert to the new information, carefully reading (and clipping!) newspapers and journals.

Find out how other people are helping young women in crisis pregnancy in your area. Discover how people in your community fight against abortion. How does your congressman vote on issues related to abortion? What churches or agencies in your area have helping programs for women in crisis pregnancy?

There's a lot to know! And as you know more, you will become a resource for other people, helping your friends and family become aware of the magnitude of the problem and the various avenues of ministry available.

Be a Friend

You've got a head start on this—you already have a pregnant friend, and that one friend may take all the time and energy you have to apply to the problem right now. But eventually you will hear of other girls—relatives, or young women in your church or community—who are thrown into this traumatic period of decision making.

Young women experiencing crisis pregnancy often find that their friends are uncomfortable around them, or that some they considered friends weren't really committed. At a time like that, a young woman is hungry for a friendship that nourishes and encourages. Dare to reach out to a girl with such a need.

Your friendship during this time says, "I don't believe in abortion and I'll inconvenience myself to help and support an unwed, pregnant friend." Remember Sandy, the very first girl who came to stay with me? Her story is in the Introduction to this book. These are her words:

While I had tremendous support from my family, I wanted to leave home for the duration of my pregnancy to spare myself and them from having to explain my condition to our local Christian community. Henrietta's home and family were evidence that God still loved me. Indeed, he provided for me beyond what I could have thought or asked. The little apartment in Henrietta's house was my hiding place, where I was neither judged or condemned. God loved me through her.

The Christian doctor and his wife were also instruments of God's grace. And the Lord provided a Christian lawyer, and a Christian counselor (Henrietta's daughter), and Christian parents for my child. I trust that God is teaching him well through them.

It wasn't easy. The day I left the hospital without my baby was and continues to be the hardest, saddest day of my life. That pain has not been equalled by any other experience to date, except perhaps the death of one I held most dear in this world.

I trust the Lord that I'll see my son again, if not before my death, then after, and I look forward to that day with joy. I wish that every girl in my situation could have a friend like Henrietta. I knew my pregnancy was a result of sin. I didn't need condemnation, but a place where I could see the consequences through. If the church is serious in its stand against abortion, then it could sorely use more Henriettas.

Clothes

Usually young women who didn't plan to be pregnant don't shop for maternity clothes with enthusiasm. In fact, many try to save every penny for use after the baby comes. Others are in school, without steady incomes of their own. Those girls who are planning to release their babies for adoption naturally don't want to purchase a lot of maternity clothes that they won't wear again perhaps for years. They can benefit from hand-me-down maternity clothing, or maybe one nice outfit or blouse that makes them feel "pretty" and cared for.

Maybe you have maternity clothes that could be loaned or donated. Or maybe you have friends who might be willing to give some things away. This is a great way to help someone in a crisis pregnancy situation.

Pregnant girls who are planning to parent their children alone will be in tremendous need of baby clothing and of baby playthings and equipment. They typically have limited budgets to work with. Any baby clothes you can collect will be a great start for these young mothers.

Finding Work

A pregnant young woman may need "something to do" during her pregnancy, especially if she left school or moved away from her home area for the duration of her pregnancy.

Babysitting is one good avenue of work for a pregnant young woman. Not only does it bring in some money, but it also gives her a better understanding of what parenting entails.

A creative friend of mine has provided hours of work for various girls who have stayed with me. She has them stuff, address, and sort various mailing projects for local businesses.

Maybe you know of someone who needs temporary help with some other kind of work—at an office, at a business, or in a home. Be creative! The possibilities are endless.

Work makes an important contribution toward how a person feels about herself. Maybe your friend or another young woman *needs* to work during this crisis time in order to bolster her battered self-esteem and to keep her growing and moving forward.

What About Your House?

Do you have an empty bedroom you are keeping warm? For whom? Consider using it for the Lord. Keeping a pregnant girl for four or five months is not a large, long-term commitment. And she might be blessed through the influence of your Christian home, your God-honoring marriage, and your church. You may be given the blessing of helping her shape some guidelines and goals for her future. And a childless home may be blessed with the unborn child being nurtured in your home.

Maybe the words of one of the young women who stayed at my house will encourage you if you are considering this direction of involvement:

I felt so alone when I found out I was pregnant. I couldn't tell my friends, and I had no one else to confide in. I was pretty sure that Jesus hated me and that there was no way he could ever forgive me.

My parents were very understanding. I had decided from the very beginning that I was going to give up the baby, and my parents agreed that this was the best decision for both me and my baby.

I didn't want anyone except my family to find out, so we looked for adoption agencies outside the city where I lived, and preferably even out of state. Through the advice of a Christian friend and counselor, we found out about the agency Henrietta works with. Although I didn't want to leave my home, friends, and family, I had no other options.

The first thing I noticed when I arrived at Henrietta's was the beautiful scenery around her wonderful home. On several occasions we saw wild deer, gophers, Canadian geese, and red foxes. Henrietta welcomed me in, and I felt very secure even though I was hundreds of miles from home.

While I was there, another girl came to stay with Henrietta. She was supposed to have her baby before me, and that helped me, too, because I could talk with someone who was in the same situation as me. We began a Bible study with some other single, pregnant girls, and we usually went out for pizza afterward. I had counseling sessions with my agency counselor every week. She helped me when I was troubled by uncertainties or just with everyday problems.

I felt like a part of Henrietta's family. I really enjoyed having her grandsons next door. We went fishing, played Monopoly, or—my favorite—King's Quest on their computer. All of her children and grandchildren were very open to me, and I appreciated that a lot.

My relationship with God *greatly* improved, and I no longer felt alone. I knew that God loved me no matter what I did.

Henrietta attended Lamaze classes with me, and when it came time for the delivery, she held my hand and stood by me every step of the way—and that was forty-nine hours.

I don't know if this letter can describe how wonderful a place Henrietta's home is, or how terrific a person she is, but I know that I made the right decision for that short time. My walk with Christ improved so much that it changed the way I felt about life before. Although it was the hardest thing to do, giving up my baby was also the most self*less* thing I have ever done.

Seeking the Lord

Maybe this time of intense friendship and interaction is an open door for sharing God's healing love and forgiveness with your friend. Even if your friend has already accepted Christ as her redeemer, she may need to be reassured of his enduring love.

Another of the girls who stayed with me talks about her relationship with God:

> Being an unwed mother is one of the most heart-wrenching experiences a young woman can encounter. I faced it as a college student, not having maintained a relationship honoring to God with my boyfriend.
>
> I was drawn through so many feelings during my pregnancy: fear, humiliation, remorse, rejection, pain, sorrow. Until the last moment I hoped to be married. I didn't want to face the pain of giving up my child for adoption, even though I felt God calling me in this direction. I struggled with the unfairness of carrying a greater weight of the burden than my boyfriend had to carry. I felt completely out of place with my peers. I was forced by the circumstances to grow up more quickly than I was ready for.
>
> But God was faithful to me. He used this time to draw me to himself. My spiritual shutters, once tightly closed, began to open. I understood for the first time God's principles for abundant life. I felt excitement about opportunities to serve him. Of course, my renewed faith didn't remove the consequences of my sin, nor did becoming obedient to God wipe away my ever-changing figure. However, the Lord walked by my side as I sought his will, and he provided for my needs.
>
> One way God provided for me was by giving me shelter with Henrietta for the last three months of my pregnancy. I needed time away from my hometown to sort through critical issues. I was tired of people's questions and longed for privacy. Henrietta's home became my sanctuary. It was there I had time to think. I had someone who listened to me and invested her time in me. Henrietta didn't have all the answers and didn't pretend to, but she helped me sift through the many questions I had. With Henrietta I felt "normal" for the first time in months. I realized I didn't have to feel disgraced forever. She and her

family made me feel at home. No one seemed to notice anything different about having young pregnant girls in this household. What a relief I felt in this atmosphere!

God provided beyond my greatest expectations. By being obedient to God's call in her life, Henrietta became a blessing to me. I am grateful for her love and encouragement. She made a tremendous difference in my life during what I consider my greatest challenge. Praise the Lord for his goodness!

Pray!

One of the greatest ministries you can have for a young woman in crisis pregnancy is that of prayer—for her and for her unborn child. Commit yourself to pray for your friend, and maybe for others who are facing the same struggle.

Also pray about your present involvement and your future involvement. Ask the Lord to open doors of opportunity for service. Ask him to give you creativity in discovering what you—with your unique gifts, talents, and personality—can do to help young women in crisis pregnancy. And then take action. God will be honored and pleased.

✳ ✳ ✳

Ways to Help

1. Read some of the books from the *Recommended Reading* list to broaden your perspective on the issues related to crisis pregnancy. Discuss them with interested friends.

2. Keep your ears and eyes open for opportunities to be a friend to pregnant young women. Or contact a helping agency and volunteer your time and resources.

3. Pray about your present and future involvement in this type of ministry. In what ways does the Lord want you to help?

Bibliography

Baker, Don. *Beyond Choice: The Abortion Story No One Is Telling.* Portland, OR: Multnomah, 1985.

Brandsen, Cheryl Kreykes. *A Case for Adoption.* Grand Rapids, MI: Bethany Christian Services, 1985.

Brandsen, Cheryl Kreykes. *A Loving Choice.* Grand Rapids, MI: Bethany Christian Services, 1988.

Condon, Guy M. *Abortion: A Crisis in American History.* Chicago, IL: Americans United for Life.

McDowell, Josh and Dick Day. *Why Wait?: What You Need to Know About the Teen Sexuality Crisis.* San Bernardino, CA: Here's Life Publishers, 1987.

Willke, Dr. and Mrs. J.C. *Abortion: Questions & Answers.* Cincinnati, OH: Hayes Publishing Company, Inc., 1985.

119

Recommended Reading

Abraham, Ken. *Designer Genes*. Old Tappan, NJ: Fleming H. Revell, 1986. Self-esteem and uniqueness are based on the fact that we wear the label of the Master Designer.

Anderson, Ann Kiemel. *And with the Gift Came Laughter*. Wheaton, IL: Tyndale, 1987. A warm and loving appreciation to birth mothers for the "gift."

Burtchaell, James T. *Rachel Weeping: The Case Against Abortion*. San Francisco, CA: Harper & Row.

Burtchaell, James T. "Women of Abortion Speak Out," *Christianity Today*, November 18, 1988.

A Dad Named Bill. *Daddy, I'm Pregnant*. Portland, OR: Multnomah, 1987.

Ezell, Lee. *The Missing Piece*. Eugene, OR: Harvest House, 1986.

Garton, Jane Staker. *Who Broke the Baby?* Minneapolis, MN: Bethany House, 1979. A brilliant disclosure of what the abortion slogans really mean. Highly recommended for family discussions with teens and pre-teens.

Hekman, Randall. *Justice for the Unborn*. Ann Arbor, MI: Servant Publications, 1984. The true story of a judge who appealed for the life of an unborn child and won.

Hershey, Terry. *Beginning Again*. Laguna Hills, CA: Merit Media, 1984. Rebuilding life after a relationship ends.

Johnson, Lissa Halls. *Just Like Ice Cream*. New York: Bantam, 1984.

Kanat, Jolie. *Bittersweet*. Minneapolis, MN: Compcare Publishers, 1987.

Kuenning, Delores. *Helping People Through Grief*. Minneapolis, MN: Bethany House Publishers, 1987.

Lehman, Dr. Kevin. *Smart Girls Don't (and Guys Don't Either)*. Ventura, CA: Gospel Light, 1982. Preparing young people to make wise decisions about peer pressure, friends, sex, drugs, dating, and more.

Lindsay, Jean Warren. *Pregnant Too Soon*. St. Paul, MN: EMC Publishing, 1988. Adoption as an option.

McDowell, Josh, and Paul Lewis. *Givers, Takers, & Other Kinds of Lovers*. Wheaton, IL: Tyndale, 1981. Bypasses vague generalities about love and sex and gets right down to basic questions.

McDowell, Josh. *What I Wish My Parents Knew About Sex*. San Bernardino, CA: Here's Life Publishers, 1987.

Michels, Nancy. *Helping Women Recover From Abortion*. Minneapolis, MN: Bethany House Publishers, 1988.

O'Brien, Bev. *Mom, I'm Pregnant*. Wheaton, IL: Tyndale, 1982.

Pierson, Anne. *Mending Hearts, Mending Lives*. Shippensburg, PA: Destiny Image Publishers, 1987.

Powell, John. *Abortion: The Silent Holocaust*. Allen, TX: Argus Communications, 1981.

Reardon, David O. *Aborted Women: Silent No More*. Chicago, IL: Loyola, 1988.

Roberts, Wes, and H. Norman Wright. *Before You Say "I Do."* Eugene, OR: Harvest House, 1982.

Roggow, Linda, and Caroline Owens. *Handbook for Pregnant Teenagers*. Grand Rapids, MI: Zondervan, 1984. A helpful guide to decision-making.

St. Clair, Barry. *Dating: Picking and Being a Winner*. San Bernardino, CA: Here's Life Publishers, 1987.

Sandvig, K. *You're What? Help and Hope for Pregnant Teens*. Ventura, CA: Regal Books, 1988.

Speckhard, Anne. *The Psycho-Social Aspects of Stress Following Abortion.* Kansas City, MO: Sheed and Ward, 1988.

Swindoll, Charles. *Starting Over: Fresh hope for the road ahead.* Portland, OR: Multnomah, 1977.

Talley, Jim, and Bobbi Reed. *Too Close, Too Soon.* Nashville, TN: Thomas Nelson, 1982. On distinguishing attraction from love.

Zimmerman, Martha. *Should I Keep My Baby?* Eden Prairie, MN: Bethany House, 1983. Direction for facing pregnancy outside of marriage.

Resources

This list is by no means complete! But I hope you will find it helpful.

Baptist Children's Home
and Family Ministries
354 West St.
Valparaiso, IN 46383
(219) 462-4111

Baptist Family Agency
Box 16353
Seattle, WA 98116
(206) 938-1487

Bethany Christian Services
901 Eastern Ave., N.E.
Grand Rapids, MI 49503
(800) 238-4269;
(616) 459-6273
   Little Rock, Arkansas
   Bellflower, California
   Modesto, California
   Denver, Colorado
   Hollywood, Florida
   Macon, Georgia
   Evergreen Park, Illinois

Indianapolis, Indiana
Des Moines, Iowa
Orange City, Iowa
Annapolis, Maryland
Wakefield, Massachusetts
Fremont, Michigan
Madison Heights, Michigan
Holland, Michigan
Paw Paw, Michigan
Stillwater, Minnesota
Jackson, Mississippi
St. Louis, Missouri
North Haledon, New Jersey
Asheville, North Carolina
Akron, Ohio
Flourton, Pennsylvania
Millersville, Pennsylvania
Greenville, South Carolina
Chattanooga, Tennessee
Memphis, Tennessee
Vienna, Virginia
Bellingham, Washington
Waukesha, Wisconsin

Christian Adoption
and Family Services
2121 W. Crescent, #E
Anaheim, CA 92801
(714) 533-4302

Christian Care Maternity Ministry
354 West St.
Valparaiso, IN 46383
(219) 465-7777

Christian Family Care Agency
1121 E. Missouri
Phoenix, AZ 85014
(602) 234-1935

Christian Homes for Children
275 State St.
Hackensack, NJ 07601
(201) 342-44235

Christian Maternity
Home Association
1817 Olde Homestead Lane, Suite H
Lancaster, PA 17601
(717) 293-3230

Crisis Pregnancy Ministries
701 W. Broad St., Suite 405
Falls Church, VA 22046
(703) 237-2100
(Contact this ministry for the number of
a Crisis Pregnancy Center in your area.)

Deaconness Home
5401 N. Portland Ave.
Oklahoma City, OK 73112
(405) 942-5001

Evangelical Child and
Family Agency
1530 N. Main St.
Wheaton, IL 60187
(312) 653-6400

Evangelical Child and
Family Agency
2401 N. Mayfair
Milwaukee, WI 53226
(414) 476-9550

Evangelical Family Service, Inc.
119 Church St.
Syracuse, NY 13212
(315) 458-1415

Highlands Child
Placement Services
5506 Cambridge
Kansas City, MO 64129
(816) 924-6565

Liberty Godparent Home
P.O. Box 27000
Lynchburg, VA 24506
(804) 384-3043

The Lighthouse
1409 E. Meyer Blvd.
Kansas City, MO 64131
(816) 361-2233

Loving and Caring, Inc.
1817 Olde Homestead Lane, Suite H
Lancaster, PA 17601
(717) 293-3230

New Hope of Washington
2611 N.E. 125th, Suite 146
Seattle, WA 98125
(206) 363-1800

New Life Homes and
   Family Services
3361 Republic Avenue
St. Louis Park, MN 55426
(612) 920-8117

Plan Loving Adoptions Now
P.O. Box 667
McMinnville, OR 97128
(503) 472-8452

Right to Life of Cincinnati
P.O. Box 24073
Cincinnati, OH 45224

Shepherd Care Ministries, Inc.
5935 Taft St.
Hollywood, FL 33021-4532
(305) 981-2060

Sunny Ridge Family Center
2S426 Orchard Road
Wheaton, IL 60187
(312) 668-9783

Wales Goebel Ministry
   (Lifeline Ministry)
2908 Pump House Road
Birmingham, AL 35243
(205) 967-4888